Endorsemen

"Drs. Jaffe and Diamond have also suffered ~~from longing to have a child,~~ and they relate how their own experiences have shaped them personally and professionally and have helped them address their patients' concerns and other couples with the emotional aspects of infertility. . . . Readers of *Unsung Lullabies* may find some peace of mind as they start the healing process of their sorrows and wounds as they read this excellent book on coping with longing for a child."

— Lori L. Arnold, M.D., F.A.C.O.G., Board Certified
Reproductive Endocrinologist and Infertility

"As an ob/gyn nurse practitioner, I see couples in all phases of infertility diagnoses and treatment. . . . The combined personal and clinical experience of the authors makes this a truly valuable resource. I would recommend this thorough, thoughtful book to couples in my practice, knowing it will be a great source of comfort and information."

— Lisa A. Clarke, CRNP, MSN, San Diego, CA

"As an adoption attorney, I see couples at the very end of the road. *Unsung Lullabies* has given me insight into *why* couples are so emotionally exhausted as they face their last hope of becoming parents. . . . I highly recommend this book to any and all who have experienced infertility as well as to professionals in the field."

— Susan Romer, Ph.D., Attorney-at-Law, Law Offices of
Adams and Romer, San Francisco, CA

"*Unsung Lullabies* is an insightful, sensitive, useful, easy-to-read resource for women and their partners experiencing infertility. It strikes the perfect balance between realism and hope as well as a balance between women's needs and men's. Too often men are overlooked in the whole matter. Reading this book will help men—and women—express themselves in their own voices and help the struggling couple through the turmoils they endure. Everyone who knows someone who is experiencing infertility should read this book."

— Gail R. Shapiro, Ed.M., president of Womankind
Educational and Resource Center, Wayland, MA

"*Unsung Lullabies* is an excellent read. The authors do a wonderful job capturing the complex emotions and issues involved with all aspects of infertility in a way the patient can relate to. I finally understand why I feel the way I do, and so will anyone going through it who reads this. After reading many technical and scientific infertility books, this was such a refreshing change."

—Kristy Echelberger, president of RESOLVE,
San Diego, CA

"I highly recommend *Unsung Lullabies* to anyone traveling down the difficult infertility path. No matter where one is currently in this journey, it is valuable. . . . So many times this process feels so lonely. Of the twelve years of my infertility struggle this is the first book of its kind."

—Linda Huston, president of RESOLVE, Ohio

"This book gives language to the experiences of so many couples who unite, disintegrate, or just drift apart when challenged with infertility. A must-read for all (both men and women!) who have ever waited around month after month for the news they are desperately hoping to hear."

—David B. Wexler, Ph.D., author of *When Good Men Behave Badly: Change Your Behavior, Change Your Relationship* and executive director of the Relationship Training Institute

"Janet, Martha, and David share perspectives that can enrich our personal and spiritual lives as we struggle to weather the storms of infertility. They bring hope that we can survive the roller-coaster ride of emotions from the first diagnosis through to deciding when enough is enough and getting off the treatment merry-go-round to find peace and eventually joy again, even if parenthood may no longer be an option."

—Sandra K. Dill, AM, executive director of ACCESS
Australia Infertility Network and director of iCSi,
International Consumer Support for Infertility Network

Understanding and Coping
with Infertility

Unsung
Lullabies

Janet Jaffe, Ph.D.
Martha Ourieff Diamond, Ph.D.
David J. Diamond, Ph.D.

St. Martin's Griffin
New York

SKOKIE PUBLIC LIBRARY

UNSUNG LULLABIES. Copyright © 2005 by Janet Jaffe, Ph.D., Martha Ourieff Diamond, Ph.D., and David J. Diamond, Ph.D. All rights reserved. Printed in the United States of America. No part of this book may be used or reproduced in any manner whatsoever without written permission except in the case of brief quotations embodied in critical articles or reviews. For information, address St. Martin's Press, 175 Fifth Avenue, New York, N.Y. 10010.

www.stmartins.com

Library of Congress Cataloging-in-Publication Data

Jaffe, Janet, Ph. D.
  Unsung lullabies : understanding and coping with infertility / Janet Jaffe, Martha Ourieff Diamond, and David J. Diamond.
    p. cm.
  Includes bibliographical references (p. 265) and index (p. 269).
  ISBN 0-312-31389-6
  EAN 978-0312-31389-0
  1. Infertility—Psychological aspects. 2. Childlessness—Psychological aspects. I. Diamond, Martha Ourieff. II. Diamond, David J., Ph. D. III. Title.

RC889.J33 2005
616.6'92'0019—dc22   2004063282

First Edition: June 2005

10   9   8   7   6   5   4   3   2   1

616.6920019
J

*This book is dedicated to our families,
past, present, and future.*

Contents

Contents

Acknowledgments

There are many people we would like to thank as we complete this journey: our literary agent, Betsy Amster, who has guided us, prodded us, and kept us company throughout every stage of this book; Jane Rosenman, for her early support of the book; Hope Dellon, our editor, who picked up the torch and has steered us through the process with wisdom and assurance; Robin Michaelson, for her boundless enthusiasm, and for pushing us always beyond what we thought we could do; Laura Bellotti, for her perceptive editing of the proposal; and Ann Harris, who has been a wonderful mentor from the very beginning. Also, we'd like to thank our families and friends—you know who you are—for their unwavering love, support, and good meals. Finally, we'd like to thank our many patients, who have shared with us the sad and happy chapters of their own reproductive stories, and from whom we have learned so much.

Introduction: The Wish to Become a Parent

When you decide to have a child, the wish to be a parent becomes almost primal. You decide to stop using contraception, start lovemaking, and imagine that conception will take place in a mystical, romantic sort of way. You begin to hum the lullabies that you've always dreamed of singing to your baby.

What you don't wish for—or even imagine—is that this won't happen. That instead of making love you might be having timed sex on a doctor's orders, giving yourself injections, providing sperm samples. What's supposed to be natural has now become a high-tech pursuit. Even if you knew or vaguely worried that you might have fertility problems, you never imagined that this would be what it took to try to make a baby.

Each of us has a story, a dream of what it will be like to become a parent. Although everyone's story is unique, we all expect our dream to come true.

But if you are brave enough to pick up this book, you know, unfortunately, that not all stories go that way. We, the authors, know this too, because our stories did not go as we had hoped. In our dreams to become parents we didn't think we'd have to utilize assisted reproductive technology either. Yet all three of us have experienced the struggle of infertility; infertility has affected each of us in unique and profound ways.

We know, all too vividly, about feeling envious of pregnant couples and then feeling ashamed of our jealousy. We know about feeling numb, angry, out of control, lost. We know the nagging worry that our spouse would stop loving us because we couldn't have a baby. We know the feeling that we've done something wrong, that somehow we are being punished. We know the craziness and loneliness infertility brings.

Who are we? First we are a married couple—David and Martha—and Janet, married to Jules. We are also colleagues, a trio of clinical psychologists who founded the Center for Reproductive Psychology in San Diego. We joined together seeking to help people, because we know what it's like to struggle through infertility without any support—that's what happened to us. And we work with hundreds of women and men, counseling them on how to deal with the emotional upheaval when their stories don't go as they hoped, whether they are coping with infertility, miscarriage, premature birth, postpartum adjustment, or other reproductive trauma.

Unsung Lullabies grows out of our personal struggles with infertility, which have shaped who we have become personally as well as professionally, and from listening to the heart-wrenching stories of the individuals and couples with whom we have worked. Their pain is our pain, and our solutions have, we hope, been their solutions. In these pages, we hope that you, too, will find insight and understanding as to why being unable to have a baby can cause an ongoing current of emotional repercussions. We believe that once you comprehend the full psychological meaning behind the labyrinth of feelings which infertility creates, you will be able to hear your *unsung lullabies*—those innermost thoughts and feelings about your longing for a baby that well up, softly at first, then more insistently, from the deepest parts of your being—without falling apart. We hope that these insights, combined with examples from the stories of others will help you to weather the storm—and go on to make the wisest reproductive decisions for yourself, your partner, and your family.

Who We Are

Before we go any further, we'd like to share some of our personal experiences. While our diagnoses differed and we underwent different aspects of the assisted reproductive technology (ART) process, we did live through similar emotional pain and trauma. And those underlying emotional similarities in our experiences far outweigh the differences in our specific individual trials.

For each of us, the way things went was painfully different from what we had envisioned and hoped. Here are our stories:

Janet

As a young girl, I loved to dance for hours and hours as "Tina the Ballerina" played on our living room's record player. Not only did I love the music, I loved Tina's story: she travels to Paris to see the ballet and saves the day by dancing the lead role when the prima ballerina is injured.

I took ballet to be like Tina. And I loved my dance classes. But

I also became very nervous when my turn came to pirouette across the room. Would I shine and get noticed for my dazzling grace and form like Tina? What would happen if I failed?

Fast-forward several decades. I married Jules in my mid-twenties, and we postponed having a baby, both busy with our careers and not ready yet for parenthood. When my biological clock chimed in my early thirties, I was surprised and overwhelmed. It was all I could do to not start designing the baby's room right away! I pictured myself dancing around the living room again—this time with a baby in my arms.

But I was also scared. The same nervous anticipation I had felt in dance class returned. It was our turn to try and have a baby and I was thrilled, but could I really do this? I worried about "being" a parent; I didn't expect to have problems "becoming" a parent.

Needless to say, becoming a parent didn't go smoothly. After my first miscarriage, I was told by various medical professionals, as well as family and friends, to "go on vacation, relax, don't think about it." I tried. I really tried. We did go on vacation and I lay on the beach, pretending to have a good time, trying my best not to think about it. Easier said than done.

My second miscarriage occurred five months later. I'd go to the bathroom constantly to check for blood during the ten weeks I was pregnant; when I started spotting, my deepest fears were confirmed. I was devastated.

As each month and each unsuccessful cycle passed, I became more and more despondent. Everyone else around me was pregnant, or it seemed that way. Conversations with other women inevitably turned to babies; I had nothing to say. I felt lost and unsure of myself. Unlike the young dancer in command of her body, my body was no longer responding the way I wanted it to. Having a baby was out of my control.

After five years of continued trying, meeting with eight different doctors, having test after infertility test, drug treatments, and surgical procedures, I had my third miscarriage. My husband and doctor, although upset by the miscarriage, were weirdly elated—I was able to get pregnant, they cheered! I could not and did not share in their excitement, however, and felt only doom. Lying on the gurney that time there was no anxious anticipation waiting for my turn. I knew the routine all too well. I felt as if I would never have a baby, and the physical pain I was feeling was nothing compared to my heartache.

Martha

When I was growing up, our family spent summer vacations camping. I loved searching for the right campsite, hiking through meadows, and roasting marshmallows around the fire. During those times I remember feeling such a strong sense of family. I always knew that I would want my own family one day, and that when I grew up, whatever I chose to do would have to be compatible with being a mom.

When I met Dave, and realized that he felt the same way, I knew a family was in our future. We agreed that I would finish my doctorate and work for a while so I could then cut down to part-time once we had children. That was our grand plan.

When we decided to begin trying, I went to my doctor and got a clean bill of health. I had always taken good care of myself. The doctor even remarked that I had a great build for carrying a baby! I stopped taking the Pill and waited the requisite three months. I was ready. Sometimes I found myself window-shopping for baby backpacks and off-road strollers as I daydreamed about when our new family would go camping.

Only nothing happened. I never got my period after going off the Pill. And when I finally did, my menstrual cycles sometimes lasted six weeks, sometimes ten.

And so our infertility journey began: months and years of taking my temperature every morning, painful tests, diagnostic surgery, shots, shots, and more shots. We even coped with diagnostic errors—one doctor told us that Dave and I were allergic to each other—which turned out not to be true and only added to our despair. How could this be happening? It was never supposed to be this way. It just wasn't fair. With each step, I felt further and further away from the family campsite I had always dreamed of.

It wasn't fair for Dave either. Although different things touched us, and different images kept us awake at night, we were both struggling with our infertility. Sometimes we could help each other and sometimes we couldn't. It was a shared loneliness as we attempted to forge a trail in this uncharted wilderness.

Dave

I've always been a fix-it kind of guy. Like my dad, I have a garage full of tools, and since working alongside my father when I was young, my favorite Saturdays have been spent tinkering with the car and working on projects around the house. I like making things, and I always had visions of building the perfect tree house, with my kids hammering away next to me. I even worried about when my kids would be old enough to use power tools. But that was before the infertility, before our project of building a family began to change.

When we first started going through it, I thought my main job was to take care of Martha; she was going through so much and I needed to be strong for her. The realization that the situation was hard for me too struck home when my friend Steve asked me how things were going. I appreciated his question, because the treatment had by this time become a major focus of our lives, and inside, I was worried about our current treatment cycle and whether it would work.

However, not wanting to reveal how concerned I was, I told Steve I was getting to be a pro at the shots, and joked that while the nurse said I should imagine poking an orange, I thought of my wife more as a peach. Steve laughed, then turned serious. "Don't tell Martha, because it might upset her . . ." he told me, as he launched into a story of a friend of a friend who had gone through a successful IVF treatment, only to lose the baby late in the pregnancy.

Steve didn't notice as I drew in a tense breath. It was neither the first such tragic story I had heard, nor would it be the last. But what hit me the hardest was Steve's opening: "Don't tell Martha, it would upset her." What the hell did he imagine it would do to *me?* I was shocked, and I was angry.

At that moment, I realized that I felt every bit as upset by Steve's story as he worried Martha would be. I wondered why people, including myself, assumed that just the woman felt the pain of infertility. What about the man? What about me? I guess it didn't occur to Steve to tread lightly with me; it was as if my feelings were invisible. After all, we were both guys. He didn't think I'd be anxious and worried too. Or even scared. But I was. Not only was I *not* invisible, but my own feelings were every bit as complex and deeply felt as my wife's.

Just like Martha, I had so looked forward to being a parent. I couldn't wait to be a father, to take care of our baby. As a kid, I had helped my mother take care of my two much-younger brothers. So I knew what to do. This added to my own pain in encountering infertility—the prospect of *not* having children was profound. I felt less manly because I could not "fix" this problem.

The Center for Reproductive Psychology

Over the years, as the three of us sat down and compared notes about our experiences, we realized how much we had in common despite the differences in each of our stories. We agreed that some doctors had been great; others had filled us with false hopes and a condescending "there, there dear, everything will be okay" attitude that was dismissive of our suffering. Other doctors seemed aggressive and wanted so much money that we retreated in helplessness. Friends and family wanted to help, but they didn't know how. As we talked, we realized how much we had all suffered as individuals and as couples, and how alone we had felt.

When we were going through infertility, there was so little support for what we really needed—a deep understanding of why it hurt the way it did, and a reassurance, whether we had a baby or not, that we would somehow survive this living hell. It has been part of our mission to provide the help that we so sorely needed. To that end, in 1996 we established the Center for Reproductive

Psychology to help others who suffer from infertility and other reproductive traumas. Unique in its focus, the center offers counseling to individuals and couples who are experiencing infertility, miscarriage, premature birth, multiple and complicated births, as well as postpartum adjustment problems. We also help people grapple with the complicated decisions regarding the use of donor technology, surrogacy, and adoption.

We also serve as a resource and educational center, with doctoral students researching many psychological aspects of reproductive issues for both men and women. Research at the center is leading to a deeper understanding of the psychological impact of infertility and other reproductive crises. We lecture nationally and internationally, at hospitals, doctors' offices, and professional conferences to increase the sensitivity of the medical community to the depth of the trauma that infertility patients are experiencing. We speak to nurses, midwives, and book clubs; we talk to whoever will listen about the importance of understanding the meaning of this experience for individuals, couples, and extended family.

Why We Have Written this Book

Not only do we lecture wherever we can, we also listen—to our clients, their spouses, their doctors, and our own hearts. Hearing our clients' stories over the years—the painful emotions and sense of isolation, the feelings of shame and self-doubt—all the feelings that we, ourselves, wrestled with, made us want to provide you with the help we didn't have.

Sadly, the number of infertile couples is staggering. According to the American Society for Reproductive Medicine, infertility affects 6.1 million American women and their partners—approximately one in ten of the reproductive-age population. More and more people are utilizing ART every year.

Reproductive technology is both a gift and a burden. On the one hand, with the incredible advances in reproductive medicine, couples have opportunities they would not otherwise have. The same technology, however, creates painful and complicated choices that people have never had to face before. *Unsung Lullabies* helps couples understand and sort through these difficult dilemmas.

We hope that the stories of our clients that we share will help you feel less alone. (Please note that to protect our clients' confidentiality we have changed names and identifying details in our case studies.) You are not the only one hurting this way, although it often feels like it.

Roadmap to *Unsung Lullabies*

In part I, we explain why we define infertility as a trauma, and how important it is that you recognize it as such. Infertility involves many painful feelings—but the experience also taps into the deepest layers of our identities as human beings, and may trigger a sense of loss and trauma that is confusing, complex, and difficult to navigate. We explore what happens when things go so wrong—how you are derailed by the medical interventions used to diagnose and treat infertility as well as the emotional side effects. We also introduce the concept of your "reproductive story," your vision of what it will be like when you become a parent. This inner narrative fuels the intense emotional issues at the heart of infertility.

In part II, we explore why all this "hurts so bad." You may feel debilitated by your diagnosis; your sense of self may be crumbling. By recognizing and acknowledging the many losses infertility causes—from the loss of feeling healthy and normal to the loss of feeling life is in control—you can gain some control over the overwhelming pain and confusion you may be experiencing.

We also focus in depth on how infertility derails your relationships with your partner and your family, with suggestions on how to cope with these changes. We also discuss the particular ways that men deal with this loss and trauma, as well as its impact on the couple. Too often the pain men experience isn't acknowledged, yet men are just as prone to intense feelings about infertility as women.

In part III, we talk about the necessary steps of grieving and how best to cope with an infertility-insensitive world. How do you acknowledge and handle the tremendous loss you feel when you get your period each month or an in vitro fertilization (IVF) cycle fails? You've invested so much personally, emotionally, physically, and financially, yet the outside world doesn't recognize your loss. Being in the world can be tricky when you feel so vulnerable. Well-meaning remarks can "zap" you; we suggest how to handle those trying situations. We also discuss how to cope with holidays, extended family, and the strain on friendships.

In part IV, we discuss how you rewrite your reproductive story as you proceed through treatment. We cover the decision of knowing when to stop trying, and how to make decisions regarding donor technology, surrogacy, adoption, and remaining childfree. We've also included a chapter on parenting after infertility, since infertility trauma can persist even after the birth or adoption of a baby.

Writing *Unsung Lullabies,* as heartbreaking as it has been at times for us, has also contributed to our own healing. We hope it contributes to yours as well, even though at times it may be emotionally difficult for you to read. We realize we are bringing up painful feelings and emotions at a vulnerable time, but we firmly believe that when you understand why this hurts so bad—the emotional havoc that infertility wreaks—you will have an easier time healing your sorrow and wounds.

PART I

Reproductive Trauma: What Happens When Things Go Wrong?

One

This Isn't How It Was Supposed to Be

For couples experiencing infertility, wanting a baby is a craving unlike any other. The intensity of your longing is matched only by the complexity of the emotional and medical maze you must navigate. When unexpectedly faced with the sting of infertility, would-be parents experience an unacknowledged trauma that leaves them feeling not only frustrated and angry, but sad, frightened, confused, guilty, overwhelmed, and out of control.

You may feel as though you are losing your mind, as you're caught up in a swirl of difficult feelings. *This isn't how it was supposed to be*, you think. And you wonder, *why is this happening to me?* We, the authors, wondered this too, as we were going through infertility, and these are the first questions that many of the women and men we work with ask us. "It's so hard to talk about this," said Emily, a thirty-six-year-old teacher. Makeup couldn't erase the dark circles under her eyes. "I never thought I would have problems getting pregnant—I've always been as regular as a clock. Everyone else seems to have no trouble. So what's wrong with me?

"It's also embarrassing," she continued. "Everybody asks when we're going to have kids and I never know what to say. I don't feel like myself. I feel like such a loser."

Emily and her husband Jack, a thirty-nine-year-old lawyer, have been trying for three years to conceive. Six months ago, their first in vitro fertilization (IVF) attempt failed; now they need to decide whether to try another cycle.

"We've been through so many tests, but nothing has worked," she cried. "I'm so tired of being poked and prodded and filled with hormones that make me feel awful. Financially, my parents said they could help out, but I don't want to take their money. And what if it doesn't work again? I don't know if I can take another loss. And if it doesn't work, then what do we do?"

You, like Emily, may be experiencing the emotional turbulence of infertility and its treatment. Your mind races as all you think about is your infertility. Or you may feel vague and distracted, and have trouble concentrating or remembering things. You may not be able to sleep, or you may feel like sleeping all of the time. You may cry at the drop of a hat; you may explode easily. You may worry that you are going crazy. You may feel like a failure.

You obsess about what your body is doing now or the next step your doctor recommends. Faced with complicated decisions, often involving costly medical procedures, you may get frustrated by the lack of clear-cut solutions. You are devastated one moment, hopeful the next. You feel as if you're on a roller coaster—careening from excitement to gloom, wishful thinking to devastating disappointment—only this ride isn't at all thrilling; rather, the longer you're on it, the more you feel as if your carload of emotions is about to go soaring off its tracks.

You feel all these things because you are going through a *reproductive trauma*. Being unable to have a baby as and when you had hoped is one of the most painful crises that couples confront. Clearly this is not how you thought it would be.

What Is Reproductive Trauma?

Often unrecognized as such, infertility truly is a trauma. A trauma is any event or feeling that goes beyond the range of usual human experience and is overwhelming either physically, emotionally, or both. It typically involves a threat to your physical integrity or that of a loved one. It may be the result of a single devastating event or a series of events that gradually build up and overwhelm you. As part of the mind's attempt to master the catastrophic overload, the events may be re-experienced in flashbacks, which can be triggered by anything reminiscent of the original events. Sometimes a general hypersensitivity and irritability occurs, alternating paradoxically with a sense of numbness and withdrawal. A traumatized person feels anxious, depressed, and has difficulty concentrating.

What makes the experience of infertility a trauma? The diagnosis of infertility, and the medical interventions often needed to treat it, represent a threat to our physical integrity, our sense of being healthy and whole. One of the most fundamental aspects of our physical selves is our reproductive capability. When that does not function properly, we doubt everything else. Infertility is a trauma because it attacks both the physical and emotional sense of self, it presents us with multiple, complicated losses, it affects our most important relationships, and it shifts our sense of belonging in the world.

When you are diagnosed with infertility, the world as you previously knew it crumbles. No matter where you are in your journey—trying the "old-fashioned way" to no avail, whether you have just been diagnosed, are using drugs to produce more eggs, undergoing surgery—your outlook on everything changes as you adjust to this crisis and what it means for your future and your dreams. The trauma of infertility is such that what you had taken for granted and expected is lost.

Moreover, like a soldier who must return to battle again and again, you face an accumulation of traumatic losses when, month after month, another menstrual cycle occurs, the procedure doesn't work, or an intervention must be canceled. Infertile couples constantly re-experience their loss—and are consequently re-traumatized—month after month. Not only do you react to one failed intervention, you react to the cumulative effect of all that you have undergone. The snowballing effect of all the treatment, all the trying, takes its toll.

How do you get through a trauma like infertility? As you and your partner go through treatment, you may hear, "Keep a stiff upper lip" or "If you have a positive attitude and you relax, everything will go well." The implied message in this well-meaning advice is that you should hide your feelings and not dwell on the negative. It may seem counterintuitive to rehash the details of your experience—after all, wouldn't it be better to forget all the bad things and move on? But this kind of trauma is ongoing and needs to be dealt with as you go through it. Talking about it helps.

Giving voice to your feelings gives you some relief from the trauma of infertility. Like an old-fashioned pressure cooker, it can help you let off steam by airing your worries, your distress, your sadness, your fears. If you can talk about what you are going through, with someone who is not judgmental, but is understanding and safe, you will gain more control over the trauma and be able to move forward.

The Emotional and Medical Roller Coaster

"Not a day goes by when I don't think about getting pregnant," said Kate, a thirty-five-year-old museum curator trying to conceive for four years. "I know I dwell on it too much, but I can't control my thoughts. After I ovulate, it gets even worse. I start looking for symptoms. If my breasts get tender I calculate my due date. I can't help myself, even though it has always turned out to be PMS. When my period comes, I'm crushed."

Not only did Kate's emotions yo-yo through each month, going from high to low and back again, but she also ruminated about her activity during the month—wondering if she were to blame. She continued, "Then I begin to worry, and second-guess, and doubt myself. Should I have exercised as vigorously as I did? Did I do too much by carrying that heavy load of groceries? Did I forget to take my vitamins? Maybe I shouldn't have had that glass of wine. I monitor every move I make, every month, every day. I know I obsess too much, but I can't stop thinking, 'What have I done to deserve this?' All I want is a baby; is that too much to ask?"

Being preoccupied with pregnancy and consumed with wondering whether or not you are somehow to blame is typical of this kind of traumatic experience. There are emotional highs and lows inherent in infertility trauma. Yet friends and family members, even your doctors, may not understand how upsetting all this is to you.

Traumatic as well are the medical procedures to diagnose and treat infertility, which are physically and emotionally demanding, invasive, and painful. And the results may bring more questions than answers, causing even further distress.

Having waited out the prescribed year of trying on their own, Marissa, a thirty-two-year-old wedding and event planner, and her husband Ken, a thirty-eight-year-old veterinarian, consulted a specialist for an infertility workup. The doctor recommended that Marissa undergo a hysterosalpingogram procedure.

"The doctor stood on one side of the room, the technician on the other, and I lay there feeling helpless. They chatted about the Lakers while they were injecting the dye into me," she said. "The technician yelled: 'The right one is blocked!' They seemed happy to find something wrong. But I was devastated. It was all I could do to not start bawling on the table."

Finding out her tube was blocked—that there was something physically wrong—shocked Marissa. It isn't surprising that the tech's announcement sounded so loud to her; the bad news distorted her perception, as if the news were echoing in her ears. Not only did she discover her body wasn't functioning the way she expected it should, but what she wanted most—a baby—felt that much more unattainable.

Now she was having trouble concentrating on work. "How can I be planning these happy parties," she asked, "when I am feeling so miserable? It doesn't make any sense." She became envious of the brides she worked with and what she perceived as their naivete. "They all seem so young and carefree—as if all they wish for will come true. I imagine them barefoot and pregnant in the next year or two, and it makes me so jealous."

Ken also felt jolted by the news. "Spaying and neutering cats and dogs is a part of my practice," he said. "I never gave it a moment's thought before, but now every time I do one, I think about what Marissa and I are going through. I wish I could laugh about it, but I can't. Going through all this is really taking a toll."

Every time your period arrives, every time you have another medical test or consultation, you must again face the loss of your dreams.

The Stakes Are High

While assisted reproductive technology (ART) provides hope for a dream come true, it can also subject infertile couples to even more emotional pain, more physical discomfort, and stress—in other words, more trauma.

By the time you get to your doctor's office to discuss infertility, you are already feeling vulnerable after experiencing several losses. In chapter 3 we discuss how these accumulated losses affect your self-esteem. As we discuss in chapter 4, when you decide to become a parent, you undergo a shift in your identity and adult development. When becoming pregnant fails to happen, you're faced with the loss of doing it the "normal" way. Because you have tried to conceive and have not been successful, it's understandable that you may feel depleted and desperate.

Shifting Gears: From "Normal" to Patient

The trauma of infertility is not confined just to the medical procedures you must endure, but reaches into the core of who you are and how you identify yourself. The shift in identity from healthy, normal person to infertility patient is one of the most disorienting and painful changes you might ever have to make.

When you are diagnosed with infertility, you are inducted into a club that you never dreamed you would be forced to join: the "I Can't Have a Baby Club." "But this isn't me!" people cry, "I've always been so healthy!" Although the shift from healthy, about-to-be-pregnant person to infertility patient may happen gradually as you try to conceive over "the required year of trying," the end result hits you like a ton of bricks.

Emily, who is considering her second IVF, described this shift in her sense of self when she was first diagnosed. "As I was sitting in the doctor's office I felt like I was in the *Twilight Zone*. Everything about it felt wrong. This wasn't the doctor's office I was supposed to be in and this wasn't the news I was supposed to be hearing. Instead of a warm, kind doctor telling me the happy news that a baby was on the way, I had a scientist coldly quoting me numbers and facts. It was as if I had been beamed into a parallel universe where everything was the opposite of how it should be." Three years later, it still feels unreal to her.

As you plough through the tests and procedures, try to remember that it is only a *part* of your body that is not functioning properly. But since reproduction is so inherently intertwined with your sense of self, it can be difficult to parcel out that part of yourself from the rest.

Where Do I Belong? I've Been Pregnant, but I Don't Have a Baby

We, the authors, have found through our own experience, as well as our clients', that within the club there are subgroups. Infertility trauma and pregnancy loss take on many shapes and forms, but underneath it all is the pain of loss. For example, if you can get pregnant, but not carry to term, does that mean you are infertile?

As Charlene said, "Even though I had four miscarriages, I never thought of myself as infertile. But I still have no baby. My doctor told me that because I have never carried a pregnancy to term it was considered primary infertility, even though I was able to get pregnant. I cringed when he said that. I don't want to believe it's true."

Similarly, women who have a child and then are unable to conceive again are labeled with secondary infertility. They may resist this diagnosis because they don't see themselves as infertile (nor do others), and yet the basis of their trauma is the same. They want a baby, but somehow a baby is out of their reach. For couples with secondary infertility, making the shift from "normal" to "infertility patient" may feel so dissonant with their self-concept—after all, they are already parents who have proved their fertility—that the ego blow is enormous.

Starting Treatment

When an infertility doctor suggests you consider ART—from starting Clomid or other ovulation-enhancing drugs to intrauterine inseminations (IUIs) to an IVF cycle—you'll have many questions. What drugs are necessary, how will your body react to them, which procedure is best, how much will it cost, and how many times should you try? There are many more practical medical questions that you can ask and your doctor can answer.

But these procedures also raise emotional questions that your doctor can't answer. How will we get through this, what if it doesn't work, what are the odds, what will this do to our marriage, and what does this say about me?

Starting treatment makes many feel "like a tinderbox about to ignite," as Rochelle said, about to take Clomid for the first time. The uncertainty of the situation made Rochelle, as it does for so many others, feel out of control, and added to her reproductive trauma.

Yet your partner may feel that your anxiety will hurt your chances. Ross, Rochelle's husband, needed to stay optimistic and positive. A successful pharmaceutical salesman, he was knowledgeable about drugs and comfortable interacting with doctors. "I don't understand why she's so on edge about taking Clomid. So many women do these days. I just wish she wasn't so tense. If she keeps thinking negatively, it's all bound to go wrong." Ross grew up with an alcoholic mother and learned to cover up painful emotions. His need to be upbeat and deny Rochelle's feelings was how he protected himself from his own anxiety and feelings of helplessness. As we discuss in chapter 7, regarding couples, part of the difficulty in dealing with infertility is that each person copes differently. Recognizing how you deal with the trauma and how your partner handles it can help prevent the two of you from misunderstanding each other. Accurately gauging each other's needs is crucial during this sensitive time.

Hanging in Midair: The Anxiety of Undergoing Treatments

Deciding what to do is stressful enough. Then there's the stress of undergoing treatments, which are both physically and emotionally taxing. The anxiety of whether or not this will work—if you even make it through a procedure—can exacerbate stress. You may find that tensions between you and your partner are at an all-time high. It's completely understandable that this is so.

Roberta and Scott, both in their mid-thirties, were having a terrible time in their first IVF cycle. Roberta's arms were black and blue from having her blood drawn so frequently. She winced every time Scott gave her an injection; feeling awful, his hands shook more, making matters even worse. Not only did the shots hurt, Roberta's swollen ovaries hurt her too. The daily doctor visits for ultrasounds were time consuming, drastically cutting into her workday.

Scott was also agitated about producing a sperm sample. "I kept worrying: what if I can't do this on demand? What will the doctor and nurses think? When I finally got in there it went okay. Let me tell you, there's nothing quite like a hospital bathroom to inspire romance!" He smiled. "The well-worn 'literature' in there made me realize I wasn't the only guy who had to do this, but I sure hope I won't have to do it again."

For many men, the relief of getting through the anxiety of producing a sample is quickly replaced by the worries about the results. Hearing any bad news—that your sperm count is low or that your motility is not the best—can send you into a tailspin of helplessness and self-doubt.

Other than making the decision to take the hormones and shots, infertile couples have no control over how the procedure will go. Your fertility cycle, your reproductive system, and to an extent, your future as parents are all in the hands of other people. The most intimate of acts between the two of you, once confined to the privacy of your bedroom, is manipulated by strangers in a sterile hospital environment.

Tammy, who has been trying to get pregnant for eighteen months, cried after her first insemination. "The doctor did everything so fast," she said. "I had wanted to at least hold my husband's hand or something as the sperm was injected, but there was no time. It was so impersonal. Whose baby is this anyway?"

And since you can't predict what will happen next, the treatment process is emotionally draining. Indeed, each step (particularly with an IVF cycle) can be a potential loss since it can fail at any number of places along the way. It may be that the egg quality is poor, or you don't stimulate well, or implantation is not successful. So much uncertainty can leave you with the feeling that everything is about to spin recklessly out of control—if it hasn't done so already. As Tammy described, "I feel like a fragile porcelain teacup, teetering precariously on the edge of the table."

Our Doctor, Our Last Hope

The loss of control you experience with infertility treatment increases your dependence on your doctors, which can further weaken your self-esteem and sense of your own competence.

As noted, Ross was far more trusting of his infertility doctor than was his wife Rochelle. For Ross, their doctor stood high on a pedestal. His view of their doctor as all-knowing provided him with relief and a sense of hope. "How can we have negative feelings about the very person who is holding the key to our dreams?" he asked. As with his alcoholic mother, he wanted to believe that all was well. He felt responsible then, as now, for keeping the emotional ship afloat.

But for many there are mixed feelings. Tara felt very attached to her doctor—he was a sensitive and caring man who was genuinely invested in helping her make a baby—but at the same time, she felt frustrated at her need to rely on him. After a failed procedure, Tara didn't think her doctor really understood. "He seemed so aloof when he called with the results—like I was just another case he had to deal with. I can't afford to get angry with him, because without him, I don't have a chance," Tara said. What Tara didn't understand was that her physician was likely having his own feelings of loss about the unsuccessful cycle.

Infertility doctors can be a complicated mix of artistry, altruism, science, and business. Most are devoted professionals who want you to get pregnant as much as you do. Since you depend on their expertise, you may idealize your doctor and his/her staff— you may look to them as having all the answers, but it is important to remember that they are just people too.

These medical procedures may be routine for your physician, but they are not for you. Infertility treatments are stressful, physically and emotionally. Your doctor is concentrating on the physical components of your treatment, not necessarily the psychological ones. Although you might want your infertility doctor to pay attention to all aspects of your care, including your emotional needs, that may be beyond the scope of his/her expertise. This can leave you feeling disappointed and even more diminished—less important—than before.

It is okay to be angry with your doctors. They may make mistakes and may not be as sensitive as you would like. Tammy's complaint that her doctor did her insemination too fast—she had wanted to hold her husband's hand—is a perfect example of how your vision of how things should go may differ from your doctor's focus on the medical procedure. If there are specific things you know you want or need from your doctor, it's reasonable to ask for them. Tammy let her doctor know she was disappointed. "Afterward, when I finally calmed down, I gave him a hard time," she said. "I teased him and asked if he had a hot date he was rushing off to. We agreed that next time we did an insemination, I'd remind him to include my husband; he was fine with that."

Because you are obliged to place so much hope in your doctor, your anger or ambivalence toward him/her can be very disconcerting. But don't be afraid to discuss your feelings with your doctor or staff. You can let them know if you disagree with them, or if you feel rushed or misunderstood. It's perfectly okay to ask questions and, if you don't understand, ask them again. It's also valid to get a second or even third opinion; you are, after all, making an enormous investment of time and money, to say nothing of your emotional commitment to this. Your doctor will not fall apart if you decide to consult with someone else. It can help to remember, whatever facility you decide to use, that the medical staff is working for you—you provide their paycheck and you are also one of their main referral sources. You are a valuable customer, and should be treated as such.

The Procedures: The First Two Weeks till Ovulation . . .

You get your period. A new cycle begins. "I am my ovaries," you think, as you wonder how many eggs you will produce this time, or if they will be any good. You feel hopeful once again. But as ovulation gets closer, your nerves become more frayed. Whether you start taking drugs for an ART procedure or wait to start self-testing for ovulation, it's easy to become hyperaware of what's happening in your body. You wait for your temperature to go up. You run to the bathroom to check if there's a change in your mucus. And, if you are taking meds, you may not feel physically well, as the stimulation makes you bloated and uncomfortable or gives you a headache and may even make you feel you are pregnant when you are not.

There is also the pressure of frequent doctor visits to monitor your progress. While the ultrasounds to see how your follicles are developing can be fascinating, it can also be stressful.

"It is exciting to watch," Lynn said. "But what if I don't make good enough eggs? Here I go again, worrying about stuff I can't control. But I mean, this is my body and yet this is happening to it. It feels so out of my control. I feel detached, like someone else is in charge, and yet so invested."

With each cycle, you become even more invested in the result. And more worried about whether or not it will work. It may feel as if your entire future is riding on this one single function of your body, of which you have no control. And as each cycle passes, you may feel more and more desperate.

It's that Time

You're ovulating, you're nervous, it's that time. What should be an enjoyable, loving moment between you and your partner feels obligatory. Or you may be going in for artificial insemination or egg retrieval. With bloated belly and partner in hand, you're off to your doctor's office for yet another procedure. What used to be a process that "magically" happened within a woman's body, now takes place using ultrasound, needles, test tubes, and petri dishes. With an IUI, there is no guessing; you know exactly when you have been inseminated. And with IVF, you can see the entire process of fertilization and watch the embryos grow.

What makes the medical treatment of infertility so emotionally painful is that technology provides you with an opportunity to attach in concrete ways to your baby-to-be. You not only watch on ultrasound as your eggs develop, if you are doing an IVF cycle, you see your "baby" when it is only eight cells old. The psychological and emotional attachment that you feel at each step of an ART procedure means that you can also suffer an enormous sense of loss at any point along the way when the procedure fails.

IVF allows you to witness the previously unseen processes of biology, and attachment may happen earlier and be more intense because of the visible evidence of an embryo. As much as people try not to attach—for fear of a loss—the process of attachment takes over and is very powerful. Therefore, if the procedure is not successful, the loss is that much more traumatic.

Judi and Adam, both teachers, devoted their summer break to trying IVF for the first time. After so many unsuccessful attempts with other procedures, they were thrilled when ten eggs of good quality were retrieved. The next day they found out of those ten, eight were mature and seven had fertilized. By the time of transfer three days later, three were good to go. At their transfer, their doctor was optimistic, proclaiming as he gave Judi a digital photo of the embryos, "There's your future family!" They were delighted with their doctor's enthusiasm.

Waiting: How Can a Glacier Move So Fast?

Time takes on an entirely different quality during infertility, whether you have tried making a baby the old-fashioned way or utilized ART. Indeed, the two weeks you must wait to find out if you are pregnant move at a glacial pace. The two-week wait can be filled with a mixture of hope, anxiety, anticipation, and fear—all magnified by each passing day. As you wait out your cycle, you may even have sensations that make you think you are pregnant. Phyllis, who took Clomid for the second month, remarked, "I felt so exhausted as it got closer to my period—I wanted to sleep all the time. I really thought I was pregnant."

You may worry that if you don't think positively, you might hurt your success. Your doctor may even suggest that you try not to think about it. In an undoubtedly well-meaning attempt at reassurance, Judi and Adam's doctor suggested they should "just go home and live life normally" after their IVF embryo transfer. But it's difficult, if not impossible, to feel "normal" or not think about it during the wait. It can help to stay busy, but know that it is also natural for you to anticipate and be on edge about the outcome.

A doctor's suggestion to not think about it runs counter to what we, as therapists—and infertility patients ourselves—have found again and again. As with most traumatic experiences, giving voice to your feelings, especially those that are negative or painful, frees you from them far more effectively than denying them. If you can speak about your emotions, you can proceed with a much clearer mind and relaxed body.

If you have delayed childbearing, the experience of time passing can be even more difficult. The doctor may look at his or her schedule and casually say, "Oh, we'll start in two months," not realizing that two months can feel like forever. The hope that time can be extended indefinitely as you pursue a career or other activity is dashed when you realize that the clock is running out and every week, every month, and every year becomes critical. It is no longer trivial to wait two weeks, to say nothing of two months.

Infertility patients know all too well, however, that even as time slows down during some phases of treatment, at others, things move altogether too fast. You go to what you think is a consultation, and the doctor suggests that you could be inseminated that day, or wants you to begin medication tomorrow. It can feel overwhelming, yet if you decline, weeks may pass before you have another opportunity. You also worry that if you don't act immediately when a recommendation is made, the doctor will disapprove, or be angry. And then where would you be—you must have the doctor's support if you are even to hope you'll get pregnant.

Finding Out

As you wait for the day your period might arrive or go to your doctor's office for a pregnancy test, the anticipation can be nerve-wracking. So many women describe endless trips to the bathroom to check whether they are bleeding. Others confess they have taken pregnancy tests before the two weeks are up. It's an agonizing time—whether you are waiting a few hours to hear from your doctor's office or even two minutes to see if your at-home pregnancy kit has turned positive—it feels as if your entire life is on hold until you know one way or the other.

Judi sobbed when she got the call. "Adam and I both stayed home all day—just waiting. I didn't know what to do with myself. I just sat by the phone, but then when it rang, I couldn't pick it up. Adam took the phone call. I could see on his face that it was a no go. The eggs looked so good, though. I was so sure that I was pregnant. I had to be. . . ."

Judi continued to cry. "The doctor said I wasn't technically pregnant, but I *had* been pregnant, even if it was just for a moment! I feel like someone has died."

So often, this is a loss that goes unrecognized. Until recently, there was not even a name for such a loss. We know, however, that this "pre-carriage," or "pre-implantation miscarriage," can be emotionally devastating. During ART, you have experienced a "pregnant moment." If it fails, it is a baby—your baby—who has died, even if a medical pregnancy was never established.

Getting Through it

Acknowledging that infertility is a trauma, no matter what stage of treatment you are in, is the first step in getting through it. Your losses are real. Even if you know that your odds for successful treatment are low, you will still be grief stricken if that treatment fails. Your reactions and feelings not only make sense, but are expected and unavoidable. To defuse the intensity of your emotions, it's essential that you explore and talk about them.

The next step is understanding *why*. The following chapters explore the many reasons why infertility is a trauma. The first of these is that infertility does not merely represent a recent failed pregnancy, but a whole lifetime of dreams, hopes, and plans that have gone horribly awry.

Two

Your Reproductive Story

My mother was a teacher, and ever since I was little, I always knew that's what I would be too. I figured it was the perfect job for a mom, having summers off and basically the same schedule as my kids. So here I am, a teacher, just like my mom, just as I had planned, only we've been trying now for five years and still no baby. —Cheryl, infertile five years

Did you plan how many kids you'd have? Imagine what their names would be? Decide whether you'd stay at home or after maternity leave return to work? Even if you hadn't decided on names yet, we all have an idea of "how it's supposed to be" when it's our turn to get pregnant and have a baby. Now that it's been so difficult to have a baby, it may be excruciating to think about your eager plans and innocent hopes when you first started on your journey to parenthood.

What Is Your Reproductive Story?

Your reproductive story is an unconscious narrative that begins in childhood and runs through your adulthood. It is your story of how you think your life as a parent will unfold. You begin "writing" your reproductive story when you are a child, and it continues to be modified and "rewritten" as you become an adult. That your story isn't unfolding as you hoped it would explains, in part, why infertility is so emotionally painful.

Each of us has a unique reproductive story. The conscious parts of this narrative can be specific—as noted above, you may already have picked names or decorated the nursery in your mind. Sometimes there is no narrative; instead, we have a picture—or series of pictures—that we don't even put into words. For example, you may picture yourself watching your kids through the kitchen window as they play together in the backyard, imagine yourself throwing a baseball to your daughter or son, see yourself sewing Halloween costumes, or hear yourself singing a lullaby to an infant falling asleep in your arms. Such images are like silent videos, or snapshots without captions—but they are imprinted in our minds as clearly as any camera could capture. These conscious images and ideas also have a subtler prologue, which consists of our interactions with our parents since we were very young. You might notice this aspect of your reproductive story in the way you have always felt comfortable around groups of children, in your doubts about whether you'd ever grow up sufficiently to take care of them, or in your image of yourself as a nurturing person.

When your reproductive story goes as planned—when there are no hitches on the path to parenthood—you're not usually aware that it exists. Only when something goes wrong—when infertility, miscarriage, or other reproductive crises force you to edit your reproductive story—can you recognize its impact. It may feel extraordinarily painful to examine your ideas and feelings about parenthood right now, when you feel so far from becoming a parent. But we've found, both personally and professionally, that when you are experiencing infertility, it's crucial to excavate and examine this story and pay careful attention to both its conscious, readily accessible chapters, and to its earlier, subtler prologue. When you begin to understand how this uniquely written story functions in your life, you'll be better prepared to deal with the unexpected and traumatic narrative you are now living through.

What the reproductive story means, how it develops, and most importantly, what happens when the reproductive story doesn't unfold as you originally envisioned, are crucial elements of infertility trauma. The clash between your lifelong dreams of parenthood and the daily nightmare of infertility is, in part, what makes infertility so devastating.

How it Was Supposed to be

As a first step to uncovering the reproductive story, we ask our clients to share with us the story of "how it was supposed to be." We want our clients to move this story into the foreground, rather than the background, of their lives.

Some clients find their stories readily forthcoming. They have thought about having children for a long time and have a vision of how their story will unfold. "I always wanted to be a parent," recalled Laura, who has been trying to have a baby for over a year. "I used to play house for hours and I would rock and feed all my stuffed animals. My mom even got me a little cradle and she would help me make clothes for my 'babies.' "

Carly, a systems analyst for a computer firm, assumed she would become a parent when and as she wished. "I've always planned to have kids. It was something that was a given," she said.

"But I was not going to do it the way my parents did. They were too young to have kids—my mother was eighteen; my father, nineteen. They were still kids themselves, and they were always arguing about money. When I was ten they divorced. I knew that I wasn't going to bring my kids up under that kind of stress. I knew I would wait, find the right guy, be financially secure. So that's what I did. I thought I was doing all the right things, but I'm still not pregnant."

For others, the reproductive story isn't as clear. Jordan grew up thinking she did not want children. She loved to travel and developed a successful career as a travel agent. But when she reached her thirties, she changed her mind. "On an airplane trip a few years back, I read a magazine article that asked you to imagine yourself at eighty years old. Well, here I was, a world traveler, and I pictured myself as a grandma, baking cookies, reading stories, taking my grandkids on trips! All the feelings I had for my own grandma came surging up. It hit me like a ton of bricks—I wanted kids! And now that I can't have them, I want them more than ever."

Men Have Reproductive Stories too

Although it is often easier to elicit reproductive stories from women—traditionally they play with dolls, baby-sit, and are expected to be the nurturer—men have reproductive stories too, and we've heard so many poignant ones over the years. It's a mistake to think that males don't feel as strongly about parenthood as females do. Little boys fantasize about being daddies, just as much as little girls dream of being mommies. One little boy we know, Nathan, loved to learn things from his father, as he told us proudly, "I can teach my kids the same way when I'm a dad."

Sometimes boys reveal their fantasies less directly. Wielding a light saber to fight off aliens and defend his planet is a boy's way to protect and nurture, and is a foundation of his reproductive story. Boys may focus their interest on trucks, sports, or other activities that they identify with as part of being a man, but as such, their play reflects how they envision themselves as fathers. Since a boy's father is his primary male role model, he will identify with his dad, not just as a man, but also as a father.

Adult men have shared with us how they thought about future parenthood when they were children. Kevin, struggling with infertility for the past three years, remembered the arrival of his younger brother. "I was six when Alec was born, and I was so proud to be a big brother. I would help my mom take care of him by patting him to sleep. It used to worry me when he'd cry. Once he got older, we fought a lot, but I was still always watching out for him." Now Alec has a baby—and Kevin doesn't, and he feels robbed of the opportunity to take care of another child.

Dean was number four out of six kids, so his family's size shaped his reproductive story. He loved chaotic family dinners, always had a built-in team to play with, and never had to be alone. "My wife comes from a pretty large family too—she's one of five. It was just a given that we would have lots of kids," he remarked. "We have a nice house, but it feels awfully big and painfully empty right now."

Derek recalled building model airplanes with his dad when he was seven years old. "My dad and I would spend hours in the basement building models. Sometimes we'd follow the plans exactly, but other times we would come up with a different idea—we'd kind of customize it." He wistfully remarked that he hoped to have a son someday to share this kind of experience. With infertility, he was unable to produce his most precious, one-of-a-kind model.

How Your Reproductive Story Develops

Whether or not we have a child, whether or not we want a child, we still have a reproductive story. You might think that your reproductive story begins when you choose to get pregnant. But this is not the case. Even if we don't have children, we once were children, learning from and identifying with our parents. And our parents' role modeling and various cultural influences also play a role. When all this material gets pieced together, it comprises our reproductive story, which is an underpinning of our adult identity. In the next sections we explore these influences so you may understand and tell your reproductive story to its fullest.

The Story Begins

"Let's play dress up," suggests four-year-old Sarah to her best friend Tommy. "I get to be the mommy. But first we have to get married—no, *first* we have to go to college, then we get married and have lots and lots of babies."

"Okay," says Tommy. "I get to be the dad. Bye! I'm off to work now!"

Scenes like these are played out in nursery schools, kindergartens, and play yards everywhere, as young children begin the process of thinking about future parenthood. Whether they're centered on a new baby brother or sister, or a favorite doll or a pet that they help to take care of, stories and fantasies about being the mommy or the daddy pour out of children without much prompting. Rocking dolls to sleep, reprimanding a pet when he's naughty, having a "family" of trucks with a mommy, daddy, and baby truck, pretending to be a younger sibling's teacher, wielding a sword to save the kingdom from evil dragons—these childhood experiences make up the first chapters of our reproductive story.

As kids, we watch our parents with fascination, wanting to do what they do—and sometimes vowing not to do what they do. A ten-year-old will insist that he will *never* make his kid eat broccoli, while a teenage girl shrieks that she will *always* trust her kids. In either case, whether children are trying to be like mom or dad—or just the opposite—the reproductive story is being encoded into their sense of who they are and who they want to be.

Our reproductive story weaves its way through our childhood and into adulthood in a thousand ways. Remember the childhood ditty: "Mary and Johnny sitting in a tree, k-i-s-s-i-n-g. First comes love, then comes marriage, then comes Mary with a baby carriage!" Such anticipatory thoughts about future parenthood are revealed at every stage of our childhood. And when our preschoolers, Sarah and Tommy, are busy playing house, they are beginning to develop their future *parental identities*. When Sarah snuggles her baby doll or when Tommy scolds his teddy bear, they are each playing at being a parent.

Your Parents' Part in Creating Your Reproductive Story

Your experience of *being* parented is another crucial component contributing to your reproductive story. Your memories and perceptions of your relationship with your own parents become internalized as you grow up, and help you to define yourself. For example, if your parents were warm and nurturing, you will likely grow up to be a warm and nurturing adult. If they were more distant, you may either be distant yourself or choose consciously to try to be closer to others, including your children.

Your notions and feelings about parenthood essentially begin as a mirroring of what you experience as a child, and this mirroring continues to develop into stories, fantasies, wishes, and plans that you carry into adulthood. Andy, age twenty-seven, recalled how his father comforted him when he had chickenpox at age seven. "My dad would come in and read to me every night. It felt warm and cozy and made me feel a lot better. I know that when I have a baby, I'll do that a lot too," Andy said.

Not only do we identify with our parents as potential parents, we also identify with how they chose to structure their lives. This, too, becomes an important piece of our reproductive story. If our father or mother was always at work and rarely home, or one of our parents stayed at home, our ideas about work and family will be affected accordingly. What we saw our parents do (or not do) can't help but color our own choices in work and love, our interests and hobbies, and our personal style of relating to others.

"I remember when I was a kid, watching my dad in his workshop out in the garage. He was always tinkering and fixing things around the house," said Paul, struggling with infertility for three years. "I thought to myself even then, 'Someday when I'm a dad, I'll be the one to fix all the stuff.' I've learned how to fix most things, but the infertility, I'm sad to say—it's beyond my abilities."

When infertility derails our plans to incorporate our parents' choices (good or bad), we can feel quite unsettled. Melissa came into treatment because she felt her life was off track. She commented that it had always been very important to her to do things on time. In college, for instance, she had considered taking a year off to work and live abroad. But she opted not to so she could graduate with her class and not fall behind. She slowly realized that many of her expectations were based on how her parents lived. "My parents went straight through college and then got married, just like Jake and me. I guess that's the real reason I didn't want to take time off from college. I wanted to do things just as they did. We always planned to have our first child after we had been married for four years; that's what my folks did and it seemed to work well for them. We wanted to have a boy first, because I liked having a big brother. I planned to name him Ethan, my brother's middle name," she said.

In talking about her life, Melissa revealed that she and Jake had been trying to have a baby for more than five years. Overwhelmed with anxiety, she felt terribly off balance because she wasn't progressing according to her own internal timetable or her parents' example. Her parents had been so successful in her eyes that she was terrified that she would fail by following a different course.

Things that were missing or painful in your own childhood also shape your reproductive story. We all know that no one's parents are perfect. Of course, no one would want to mirror or pass on extreme cases of family dysfunction. Seeing parents fighting, witnessing alcoholism or drug abuse, or experiencing emotional, physical, or sexual abuse are not what we want for our own children. But in every family, there are less extreme behaviors that we may still want to avoid. Maybe our parents nagged us a lot, leaving us feeling unworthy or underappreciated. Perhaps they neglected to spend enough time with us or to listen to what we had to say. These are things we didn't like and don't want to repeat. So we may decide that we want to do things differently with our own children, to heal old wounds or provide something that we didn't have.

The lessons Carly learned from observing her parents shaped her choices. From an early age, she knew she wanted to make different choices from those of her parents, in her approach to both marriage and parenting. Carly never imagined she would have reproductive problems; now her despair in facing infertility is intensified by her fear that she will never have the chance to "do it right."

Many of us who had similarly troubling childhoods feel that if only we are able to do it our way with our own kids, we will be able to heal the old hurts and wounds, maybe not perfectly, but well enough. And often this *is* what happens. On the other hand, when you have counted so long on having children, and the circumstance of infertility interferes with your plan, it is difficult to recognize any other way to "fix" the past.

The Role Other Family Members Play

Your reproductive story is further enhanced by your interaction with extended family and by the experiences, stories, and memories handed down or shared between family members. Sometimes we feel that we have to measure up to how our relatives enacted the roles of mother and father; sometimes we hope to do better, but in either case these legacies—and the perceptions of them— become woven into the fabric of our reproductive stories.

Susan, trying for nine years to have a child, observed how her family influenced her ideas of fertility. "My grandparents came over on the boat at the turn of the century. They brought five kids and then had four more. They were so poor that the baby had to sleep in a dresser drawer, but their hardships did not stop them from having kids," she said. "I have forty-three first cousins from that side of the family, plus three brothers, all of whom have kids too. Fertility just didn't seem to be an issue in this family—until it came to me." Susan now feels like the black sheep of the family.

Likewise, Joanne, infertile for six years, said, "I had always been told that all the women in my family were 'built to carry babies.' I used to be so proud of that."

When you incorporate the stories your family tells you into your own reproductive plans, you may be hoping to continue the family lore. You hope that your parents and grandparents will be pleased when you emulate beloved family traditions.

You may also want to give your parents the gift of grandchildren. Not only does this further your own reproductive story, but it allows your parents to write the chapters of their own reproductive stories that contain their dreams and feelings about becoming grandparents. Fred, a retired restaurant manager who has two married daughters but no grandchildren, regretted not spending more time with his children when they were growing up. "I was so busy working and making a living; I missed out on so much. My daughters are wonderful people, but I don't think I was the best father. I'm looking forward to having grandchildren so I can have another chance at it."

Part of the pain of infertility is that it won't let you fulfill your parents' reproductive stories. You feel as if you fail them as well as yourself. But, sadly, your parents may themselves feel that they are somehow responsible for your inability to get pregnant. For example, in the 1950s and 1960s doctors often prescribed DES (diethylstilbestrol), a synthetic hormone, to prevent miscarriage.

However, women whose mothers took DES have had considerable reproductive tract damage, and more than the average share of problems with miscarriages, ectopic pregnancies, premature births, as well as infertility. (DES is now banned.) The irony, of course, is that these mothers were trying to prevent miscarriage, yet their efforts became a factor in their own daughters' reproductive trauma.

It is not only circumstances like the use of DES that make your parents' reproductive lives evident in your own. As you struggle to get pregnant, you are constantly faced with your parents' own fertility—their ability to have you—which can make your infertility feel even worse. Your own infertility can be puzzling to your parents and to yourself. You may question: "How could *we* possibly have problems having children when *their* reproductive story unfolded so smoothly?"

Or, as sixty-two-year-old Doris pondered, "I really don't understand why my daughter is having trouble getting pregnant. It was so easy having my own children. I just decided it was time and then it happened. I can't imagine why this is happening to her. I want to be a grandparent so much. When my friends get together and talk about their grandkids, I feel very left out."

Although Doris was dealing with the loss of a part of her own reproductive story, remarks like hers can be very hurtful to those of us going through infertility. (How to cope with your parents and other family members while dealing with these multiple layers of feelings and loss will be covered in chapter 9.) What is important now is to recognize that your parents have an ongoing reproductive story of their own, which continues to play a significant role in the way your reproductive story is written.

How Culture Influences Your Reproductive Story
Historical Influences

Pregnancy and childbirth have been central to our cultural experience since the beginning of human history. From the days of
the earliest hunters and gatherers, it was a man's job to go off to
"work," to protect and provide food and shelter for the family. In
part, because of the physical demands of pregnancy and breast-
feeding, it became the woman's job to take care of home and
hearth, which included caring for the young.

The gender-role differences that derived from biological imper-
atives were thereafter woven into the very fabric of society, and reflected in the history of art, religion, and mythology around the
world. Although stay-at-home dads are becoming more accepted
nowadays, the cultural stereotype that men go to work and women
raise the children still lingers. Even our preschoolers played out
this scenario. Indeed, many women who work outside of the
home still find that the lion's share of child rearing falls to them.

If the cultural expectation is that women should raise and nurture children, how does our society's prevailing ideology affect a
woman when she discovers that she can't get pregnant? How will
others perceive her?

Historically, childless women were stigmatized as barren and
abnormal. The Old Testament tells the story of Hannah, one of
Elkanah's two wives. Hannah tried for years to have a child, while
Elkanah's other wife had given him many heirs. Hannah was very
bitter about her infertility, which was exacerbated by the second
wife's constant ridiculing of her for not having children. Dis-

turbed by her infertility, Hannah went to the temple to pray for a baby (where usually only men went to make sacrifices) and poured her heart out to the Lord. Indeed, Hannah changed the nature of prayer forever after, for she was the first to pray directly to God with prayers from a grieving heart. This biblical story illustrates the pain and humiliation of infertility, and how isolated a woman can feel.

In the modern world, childlessness is still considered aberrant. Although many more women today choose to remain childless, these women may still be seen as nonconformist, unfeminine, or threatening to the continuity and well-being of our culture. When women are childless *not* by choice, they may face the same judgments by society and often experience tremendous shame, just like the biblical Hannah.

And what about men? How does our culture regard a man if he is unable to create a family for whom he can provide, thereby demonstrating his manhood? People may assume he is gay or unmanly, immature or selfish. Yet a man's longing to be a father and his wish to continue his family line are as much a part of his identity as motherhood may be for women.

Indeed, a man's sense of pressure to fulfill his societal role has altered history just as it has for women. Consider Henry the VIII of England, who struggled with many reproductive difficulties and went through six wives trying to produce a male heir. He and his wives suffered miscarriages, stillbirths, and infant deaths as well as infertility. In a sense, the Church of England was born of Henry the VIII's reproductive trauma, since he broke from the Catholic Church to give himself the option of divorce when his first wife, after many failed pregnancies and infant deaths, was able to produce only one live child, a girl. The beautiful Anne Boleyn was beheaded after she had a daughter instead of a son.

Popular Culture

Popular culture also influences how your reproductive story develops. Think about the families you saw on television shows or movies that you watched as a kid. Old reruns of *Leave it to Beaver, Father Knows Best,* or *The Brady Bunch,* for example, present idealized pictures of family life—pictures that may have shaped your image of how a family should be. Likewise, the books you read—such as *Cheaper by the Dozen*—all contribute to your internalized reproductive story. Even movies can sneak in and influence you. "My favorite movie as a kid was *The Sound of Music,*" said Annette. "I wanted to be part of that family. Julie Andrews always knew exactly what to do and say; she took care of those kids so well."

But cultural influences don't just come from the past. More recent events also shape your story. Media stories that push the envelope on age limits for parenthood make headlines, adding to our sense that childbearing should be timeless. The impact this has on your reproductive story? You may believe on some level that your biological clock will tick longer than normal. (Easy to say until you're faced with age-related infertility.) In addition, the popularity of birth-control pills, introduced to the public in the 1960s, and the era of sexual freedom that ensued, influenced the reproductive stories of most women of childbearing age today. The Pill added to our sense of control, allowing us to *avoid* pregnancy until we were ready. The unspoken message? If you're in control of when *not* to get pregnant, you can be in control of *getting* pregnant.

These cultural messages—whether subtle or blatant—have considerable impact on our lives and on our reproductive stories, even though we may not be aware of their influence until infertility hits.

Current Medical Technology and Your Reproductive Story

The medical treatment of infertility has progressed at light speed in recent years. Procedures that may have been ineffective a few years ago now have been refined to a much higher degree, presenting the infertile couple with an overwhelming array of choices and decisions.

What does the availability of so many high-tech options mean for your reproductive story? First, it suggests that you can extend your reproductive years. We have all heard of surprise pregnancies—"change-of-life babies"—that occur in perimenopausal women, but it used to be that menopause was the end of the line. Now it's possible (though still rare, difficult, and not always a good idea medically) for a woman past menopause to get pregnant and bear a child.

Technology also affects your story in terms of the sheer number of options that are available—and the time, money, and emotion you'll be investing in each one you choose. Having so many options can be bewildering yet enticing; there's hope where historically there had been none. Some advertisements for IVF clinics state that you *can* have a baby, and offer a "money-back guarantee."

However, these ads promising a baby don't necessarily tell you what you must do in order to get one. The disclaimers are never in bold type. Such hope-filled messages play on your emotions and draw you in. When there is yet another option, it can feel like you can never say no. As Tina, who has spent five years trying to have a baby, remarked: "I need to know that I have tried everything possible, otherwise I will live with regret. Our doctor has given us odds on various procedures, and I don't think we'll quit as long as there's even a small chance of getting pregnant."

Yet Tina, like you, knows that infertility treatment is not easy, glamorous, or pretty. It's an assault, it's exhausting, it's risky. And it's an enormous loss to have your efforts end without a baby. In chapter 10, we help you make choices about the future of your reproductive story: when to continue with treatments or when to say enough is enough.

Telling Your Reproductive Story—A Step toward Healing

When a person is traumatized, it is very difficult to imagine ever not feeling that way or being able to incorporate the traumatic experience into one's life. As with other traumas, the infertility trauma is marked by the feeling of being trapped.

Given that your lifelong plan of becoming a parent isn't going as intended, you may feel stuck in your tragic reproductive story—and unable to see any way out. To feel better, it's crucial that you understand how your reproductive story functions in your life.

Your reproductive story needs to be told. When our clients are able to tell their story, they develop a better understanding of why infertility hurts as much as it does. Telling your uniquely written reproductive story allows you to put infertility into the broader context of your life. It is not just the loss of pregnancy and birth that infertile couples suffer; it is also the loss of their dreams and hopes for the future. When couples share their reproductive stories with each other, they gain insight into their past, their goals for the future, and what parenthood means to each of them.

Your reproductive story may be readily accessible, or you may only gain insight into its many facets over time. The more you think about the things that have influenced your story, the more you remember about your own childhood, adolescence, and earlier adult life, the more depth it will take on. We've discussed many of the ingredients that make your unique reproductive story: your parents are likely the biggest influence, but also consider the other cultural and medical factors that we have noted.

As you ponder your reproductive story, please reflect on your thoughts and feelings about wanting to be a parent. Here are some questions to help draw your story out:

- Did you have a favorite doll or stuffed animal? A favorite story, movie, or TV show? How did they shape your reproductive story?
- When do you remember first wanting children? How many did you think you would have? Did you want to have a family by a certain age? Did you pick out names?
- What were some of your favorite things to do with your parents? Your grandparents?
- What was your least favorite memory of childhood? How does this influence your feelings about having your own children?

- What do you want to re-create about your own family of origin and the relationships you had with your parents and siblings? What don't you want to repeat?
- How is your story different or the same as your partner's?

Remember that your reproductive story is as personal and unique as you are.

The Infertility Diary

Writing Your Story

As you reflect on your past and remember stories that influence your reproductive story, it's a wonderful idea to write down these memories. We suggest keeping an "infertility diary," where you can write about your reproductive story and record the details as they arise.

Here you can record childhood memories, both happy and sad. You can write about how you would like to raise your own children, and how that may be different from how you were raised. Writing about these memories and dreams make them more tangible—and your story may become clearer so it's easier to share with your partner. It can be eye opening to discover where your reproductive stories are similar and where they differ.

Some couples choose to share one diary or you may choose to keep separate ones. Whatever you choose, remember it can be helpful to share what you discover with each other, to let your partner in on what you have written—and vice versa—so you both better understand what each other is grappling with. Writing in the diary can be an activity you decide to do together—further strengthening your bond.

If you are pursuing this journey of becoming a parent on your own, you may choose to share your story with someone close to you. Whatever your circumstance, you may find it beneficial to discuss your reproductive story with members of a support group or in therapy. Writing and talking about your story with others will help alleviate the isolation you may be experiencing.

Journaling Your Feelings

You can also use your infertility diary to vent a myriad of feelings. Journaling is a wonderful way to get things off your chest—and something you can do privately. We encourage you to track your feelings of anger, sadness, anxiety, or depression—as well as feelings of hopefulness, excitement, and happiness. You can follow events of each day or week, and learn how your emotions are likely to spill over into every area of your life. It becomes much more apparent how infertility can affect your relationships—with your partner, friends, co-workers, and family—when you can see a pattern of responses and reactions.

Daphne started keeping her infertility diary after a year of trying to conceive. "I found it helpful to write things down. Not only did this release a lot of frustration, I could also see how my mood fluctuated depending on what was happening. And there was so much going on that it started to become a big blur. Having my diary to refer to made it all so much more understandable."

Looking at her diary entries, Daphne noticed that whenever she got her period, she was more likely to argue with her husband. "This was more than just the normal PMS crankiness," she said. "I was angry. And I took it out on Sean." Seeing the pattern, she could talk to Sean about it. "I let him know it was not about him."

What it was really about was, once again, she was not pregnant. Recognizing this helped Daphne modulate and control her emotions, and Sean, now understanding what fueled her anger, was able to be more compassionate when her period came.

Tracking Your Medical Procedures

A third use for your infertility diary is to use it to keep track of your numerous medical consultations and procedures. It is extremely useful to write down in one place the dates of your procedures, your reactions before and afterward, and any advice the doctor may have given you. You can also list questions for your doctor here. And when a consult or procedure is especially upsetting, your diary can provide a constructive means to release your pent-up emotions during these particularly stressful times.

Having all this information in one place helps give you a sense of control, when it feels like all other control—of your body, your menstrual cycle, sexual relations—has been taken away.

Your Story, Your Self

Your reproductive story, whether in narrative form or as a series of wordless images, is a fundamental part of your sense of self, a cornerstone of your identity. It grows and evolves as you grow and evolve, and when all goes well, it simply unfolds as you wish it to, without your ever really becoming aware of it. In fact, it may only become a conscious story when you experience an obstacle to becoming a parent. Sometimes, it is the pain you feel—the sense of disequilibrium when faced with reproductive difficulties—that brings your reproductive story into focus.

Looking back to the beginnings of your reproductive story can help you figure out where you are now in terms of your thoughts about becoming a parent. You can clearly see that your hopes and expectations for parenthood are deeply ingrained. They are part of your core identity, part of the psychic glue that allows you to feel whole and intact. When your story fails to go as expected, when the glue fails to hold, your very sense of self is threatened.

As you go through infertility treatment, you are faced with a great many feelings, challenges, and losses. In the chapters that follow, we discuss these experiences and how to handle them. As you read, we hope that you will think about your reproductive story and notice how it changes and evolves as you progress through treatment. You may feel as if your reproductive story is being whittled away with each new intervention. You will learn to grieve each lost part of your story, and how to rewrite it along the way. Your story will always be yours and will always be a part of you. Right now you are in one of the most important and painful chapters of your life. Try to remember that it is a work in progress.

PART II

The Pain of Hope:
Why Does It Hurt So Bad?

Three

The Losses of Infertility

We are all put together, so to speak, like so many pieces of a jigsaw puzzle. When the puzzle is complete, we feel whole; our psyches are in one piece and we feel good about ourselves. If a few pieces are missing, we may feel a bit off, but otherwise ourselves; the picture of the puzzle and our sense of self are still fairly intact. But when too many pieces of the puzzle are missing or damaged, the meaning of the picture is lost and we feel confused and not ourselves.

With infertility, too many puzzle pieces are missing. Like the puzzle that loses shape when too many pieces are lost, infertility causes our sense of self to fragment. Our sense of who we are becomes undermined and weakened; rather than feeling solid and whole, we feel vulnerable and scattered, wounded, depleted, and confused, like we're running on empty. This helps explain why when someone innocently asks us, "When are *you* going to have children?" we crumble with grief.

One of the problems with infertility loss is that although we know something is terribly wrong, we can't always place a finger on what is causing so much pain and sadness. Obviously we can't have a baby, but the impact of infertility goes much deeper and shakes our very foundation. In this chapter, we focus on the missing puzzle pieces such as:

- the loss of the experience of pregnancy and birth—you long for a baby, but you also feel you are missing out on one of the most miraculous events of life
- the loss of a sense of belonging—you feel like a misfit among your friends, your family, or in society at large
- the loss of being in control—of your body, your life— your body isn't doing what you want it to do
- the loss of feeling healthy and normal—your identity shifts from "healthy person" to "infertility patient"
- the loss of feeling competent—you feel as if you can no longer achieve what you set out to do
- the loss of sexual intimacy, identity, and privacy—what had been the most private and intimate of acts is now scrutinized by doctors and medical staff

Some of these losses are obvious, and it's vital that they be acknowledged and not minimized. Other losses are less apparent, and these too must be uncovered and considered.

What we have found with our clients, as well as in our own personal dealings with infertility, is that identifying our thoughts and feelings about these losses—moving what is lurking in the unspoken and unacknowledged corners of our minds into our conscious awareness, where it can be reflected upon and perhaps shared with others—is essential to help us put the pieces of the puzzle back together again.

The Loss of Pregnancy and Birth

The most obvious loss, and the loss common to all of us who experience infertility, is that of having a baby. But even this is not a single or simple loss. Not only do we lack the baby we long for, we also are denied the physical experience of pregnancy and birth. This loss has unique meaning for each of us. The shape of pregnant women, for example, magnetized Joanne. "When I see a pregnant woman I am so envious of how big and round she is. I want it to be me! I want to feel big—even if it's uncomfortable—and know that it's because I am growing life inside me."

Kristin, after attending her sister-in-law's baby shower, felt devastated that she too couldn't celebrate a pregnancy. "My feelings were all over the place," she sobbed. "On the one hand I really wanted to help prepare all the food and plan the party. I am so happy for her. But seeing all the adorable baby outfits she got hit me hard. I don't think I'll ever get the chance to have people do that for me."

Leanne, trained as a midwife, focused more on the birth process itself. "I've watched natural childbirth a thousand times and it's still miraculous to me," she said. "To see my own child enter the world is something I long for." Her face darkened. "If we ever get to that point," she added sadly.

Skipping over these losses of pregnancy and birth minimizes their importance. We ask our clients to share with us their thoughts, feelings, and images about pregnancy and birth, and to spell out the specific things they long for. Greg, Kristin's husband, described his hope poignantly. "I have always imagined being there at the birth, video camera in hand. I even bought a new camera last year when we thought we would be pregnant. Now I feel I should return it, but that would seem like we were giving up. With infertility, you have to give up so much. But you have to feel like you can hold on to something, have some part of what you've always dreamed of."

Talking about the loss of pregnancy and birth gives you the opportunity to acknowledge what you personally long for—whether it's wearing maternity clothes, decorating a baby's room, or cutting the umbilical cord. Talking about it allows you to uncover this portion of your reproductive story, which may have been hidden away and only becomes apparent when there is a glitch in the process. What's important to remember here—and as we discuss other losses in this chapter as well—is that labeling and understanding these losses is a necessary step in the grief process. Grieving the losses of infertility will be discussed in chapter 8, but an important first step in the process is identifying and acknowledging the many losses involved.

Where Do I Belong?

"I remember years ago, when my friend Jane told me she got engaged, I sat smiling at her, expressing my congratulations, but in my mind ran a ticker tape of what's wrong with me, why couldn't I meet someone too," said Lydia, who was diagnosed with infertility two years ago. "And now when I hear the news of another friend's pregnancy, I feel the same way."

If we can't have children, how do we relate to the rest of our family, our friends, indeed, society at large? Where do we belong, we ask ourselves, if we can't have a baby? Not only is our sense of self threatened, so is our sense of our place in the community.

Abbie, a thirty-two-year-old occupational therapist in a large rehabilitation hospital, loves her practical impact on her patients' lives and her sense of camaraderie with the staff. "It's amazing to watch patients work so hard and will their bodies to function again. This kind of work calls for a team effort. I know I can count on everyone here; we are a very tight group—professionally as well as socially."

But Abbie has felt less connected with her co-workers of late. Abbie and her husband Bill have been trying to have a baby for the past two years. Six months ago she conceived, but miscarried at eight weeks. She's been despondent ever since, in part because several co-workers are either pregnant or have babies. "They seem to be falling like dominos," she cried. "Everyone is getting pregnant and having babies but me! I keep waiting—with dread—to hear who's next. It should be me, but it isn't!

"It didn't used to bother me—all these people around me getting pregnant or having babies. But now I find myself wanting to avoid their company. Gina and Lori are completely engrossed with their babies—as they should be. I don't fault them for that—but I can't handle it when they talk about poop and spit-up and who's rolling over and who's starting to crawl. I get so angry inside. I feel totally out of the loop; I *am* totally out of the loop. And then I feel guilty, like I'm uncaring or selfish. I don't know what to do or say. Last time I was with them I just sat there with this dumb smile on my face trying to be part of their world, but in reality I was desperately trying to keep from crying."

Abbie wanted to be happy for her friends, but being around

them was exceedingly painful. They had moved forward, as she had expected of herself, and she felt left behind. Not only could she not have a baby, Abbie couldn't be the supportive and caring friend she prided herself on being. Instead, she wanted to distance herself from them, but at the same time longed for their comfort and support. Confused by conflicting emotions, she felt alone. She was sad for herself, and bitter and envious of her friends—all uncomfortable, unfamiliar feelings.

Not fitting in with peers cuts to the core and makes us feel as if there is no right place for us. We don't fit into the world of parents—the world where children are such a huge focus—nor do we feel as though we belong in the realm of young couples not yet ready to start a family or those deciding to be childfree. We're in limbo, and like Abbie, we feel out of step with peers who are also of childbearing age. They are moving forward in their reproductive stories, while ours has taken an unexpected turn—into a dead-end alley. Everyone else has been invited to a fabulous party, but our invitation still hasn't arrived and we don't know why. When faced with not being invited to the "reproductive party," it may feel as if there is nothing we can do to restore our sense of belonging.

The Holiday Spirit—Where has it Gone?

The calendar year, resplendent with all sorts of social demands, provides little respite for infertile couples. Holidays, birthdays, weddings, baby showers—any and all of these get-togethers can feel like a minefield. Shelly, a librarian in her mid-thirties, described her agony of trying to decide what was worse—participating in these functions or not.

"I found myself welling up with tears as I decorated the library for Halloween. From now until New Year's, it's one family get-together after another. If I go, I am going to be miserable. Some-one is more than likely to say something that will bring on the tears," she said. "Truthfully, even if no one says anything, I'm still a mess. It's me who is thinking I don't belong because I don't have kids. But then, if I don't go, I feel as if I'm missing out."

Giving yourself a choice in these situations helps you feel more in control. Going to Thanksgiving dinner may feel okay, but going to a birthday party for a friend's one-year-old may be too much to handle. Choosing which events to attend and which to avoid puts you back behind the steering wheel and leaves you feeling less helpless. Of course, there are no clear-cut ways to handle these sit-uations; whether you attend events or not depends on your emo-tional state and how obligated you feel to go. What feels right at one moment may feel wrong at another. And it may feel like what-ever you decide, you lose out on *something*.

If you do opt to attend a social function, it helps to have some ready escape tools at hand. We advise our clients to have a signal to alert their partner that they need to leave or escape briefly in order to regain composure. We also suggest not hosting anything your-self. Although it's fine to make a cameo appearance at someone else's party, you can't escape an event at your house. You may also want to talk to your host beforehand and explain why you might need to leave early or cancel at the last minute. Of course, this strategy may not be appropriate in all situations. There are times when you will want to maintain your privacy and should, but of-ten people understand and empathize with your dilemma. There may be no perfect solution, but it does help to know you are not helpless in these situations and that you can exercise some degree of control.

I've Lost Control of My Body

What we had thought was a given—having a child—is not happening. Our bodies are not functioning the way they should; they are failing us and we are often left feeling helpless in our attempts to fix the problem. What should have been so easy has become physically and emotionally challenging. Unlike Abbie's rehab patients, who seem to will their bodies to function again, getting pregnant doesn't work that way. No matter how hard you may try, this is truly out of your control.

Erika, like so many other infertile people, expressed the irony of diligently using birth control for so many years. "When I think about all those years of birth control—all those years of trying *not* to get pregnant—I can't help but feel like I've been ripped off."

As essential as effective contraception is, it creates the illusion that bodily control is ours. After all, if we can control a pregnancy from happening, we assume the opposite is also true. Indeed, the notion that it will be easy to get pregnant is part of our collective reproductive story. The cliché, of course, is your friend or sister or cousin who jokingly, albeit proudly, announces, "All he needs to do is look at me, and I get pregnant." We have heard it so often, that when it doesn't happen for us on the first month of trying, or the second or third, we start to feel damaged and inadequate.

"I used to joke with my husband that he wasn't looking at me often enough," said Lydia. "Then I started taking my morning temperature and using an ovulation kit to make sure we did it at the right time. But that didn't work either, even though my period was as regular as could be. I'm just getting more and more mad at my body—and at me."

After months or years of trying and still no baby, the progressive sense of loss takes an enormous toll. Then, when you choose to utilize reproductive technology, you quite literally give reproductive control of your body to the infertility specialists. Your cycles are no longer natural; they are medicated and timed. The hormones you are prescribed leave you feeling tired, bloated, irritable, and depressed. What had always been a function of your own body rhythms is now controlled by medications. Your ovulation is tracked by ultrasound and the doctor "orders" you when to have sex.

It is difficult to feel so disconnected from your body. Even though you cannot will yourself to become pregnant, it is important to remember that you are in charge of decisions regarding your medical treatment. You choose your doctor, and it is up to you whether you want to pursue a particular treatment—or not. One way to get through this loss is to remind yourself that just because you are under the care of a doctor does not mean that you cease to be in charge of other parts of your life. The reproductive system—although of great import—is just one piece of who you are.

Going to the Doctor Must Mean I'm Sick:
The Loss of Feeling Healthy and Normal

Although infertility is much more common than most people realize, it never feels "normal," and also calls into question people's overall sense of their physical health.

The necessity of taking on the role of infertility patient provokes a major disruption in the sense of self. No longer able to see yourself as healthy, the other alternative is to view yourself as sick. Mary, who recently underwent a laparoscopy, said the experience made her feel less like a normal human being and more like a "case."

"I walked into the hospital wearing my own clothes. But that *me* was soon left behind. As I changed into the hospital gown, I had the sense that I was losing myself with each article of clothing I removed and stuffed into the plastic bag they gave me." Mary admitted that she was also nervous about the anesthesia and surgery, but when the nurse snapped on her hospital bracelet, she could really feel her sense of self disappear. "I was reduced to my reproductive parts and had become just another body on another gurney."

As Mary's experience illustrates, our feelings about ourselves, our partners, and our relationships change when we undergo infertility treatment. Shifting from her previous sense of self as healthy and competent, Mary now donned the label of "infertile woman," which filled her with shame, like a scarlet "I" attached to her forehead.

The loss of feeling healthy and normal can also reawaken past worries about our health and our bodies. Dale, a thirty-eight-year-old man who suffers from a low sperm count, noted, "I remember as a teenager, we would kid each other about 'shooting blanks.' Everybody always laughed a lot, but inside, I secretly worried. What if I didn't have what it takes? And then it turned out to be true." For Dale, the diagnosis of infertility confirmed old doubts about his adequacy as a man.

Becoming a patient can be an enormously disorienting and psychologically uncomfortable event. Again, it is critical to your sense of well-being to be able to separate the piece that is "infertility" from the rest of your identity. We encourage you, as we do our clients, to remember that you are more than just your reproductive parts. Although the loss of feeling healthy and normal is profound, if you can keep that loss separate from the rest of who you are, it will be easier to cope.

Loss of Feeling Competent

The inability to have a child often makes otherwise very capable people feel inept at everything. Leslie, a usually upbeat kindergarten teacher who has struggled with infertility for a year, lost faith in her abilities—not only in having a child, but in the workplace as well. "I used to be so good at keeping the kids interested and involved, and I usually can use humor rather than punishment to help them maintain their good behavior," she said. "But I feel like the class is out of control. Everyone is interrupting, talking back, and squabbling. Now, not only is my body not working right, even my classroom is falling apart."

Distracted by the onslaught of emotions triggered by infertility, Leslie lumped together the loss of feeling whole and intact with her classroom experience. Her loss of faith in herself as healthy and competent spilled over and tarnished her view of herself as a great teacher.

For Leslie, as with so many of our clients, keeping infertility separate from the rest of her life was extremely difficult, but it was an essential component of her feeling better. In chapter 5 we talk more about how to *compartmentalize,* or keep separate, one part of your emotional self from the rest of who you are. But for now, keep reminding yourself that "infertility is only a part of me; it's not all of me." You are competent in other areas of your life.

Sex Just Isn't Sexy Anymore: The Loss of Sexual Intimacy

Rick, a thirty-seven-year-old man who has been struggling with infertility for three years, spoke of another painful infertility loss. "Does anyone understand what it feels like to wake up every morning to the obnoxious 'beep, beep, beep' of a thermometer? What happened to spontaneity—and to soft lights and romantic music as a prelude to sex? I feel so bad for my wife, having to go through this ritual. And I can't believe I'm saying this, but there are times when I don't enjoy having to have sex. Sex just isn't sexy anymore."

It is very hard to feel romantic when a woman looks at her partner and all she can think of is: Are those sperm in good shape tonight? Did he wear his boxer shorts to keep everything cooler? Or he thinks: Am I on duty tonight? Will we be in the mood?

Although the initial efforts to make a baby can improve or increase a couple's sex life, infertility can disrupt sexual activity and desire. The regimentation of sex caused by infertility can interfere with spontaneity and enjoyment. Waiting until you are in the mood does not work. Planning some time for recreational sex with your partner can help, but it also may feel strained. Sex as an activity other than baby-making may feel foreign and pressured.

The loss is not just about sexual intimacy, but can also extend into the heart of the relationship itself. Perhaps it's because our partner is a constant reminder of our loss, but it is ironic that the very person we need the most at this time turns out to be the person that we get angry and frustrated with, and can't stand to look at anymore.

Mark and Sheila, a couple in their mid-thirties, started therapy because Sheila, a very down-to-earth, pragmatic graduate student in chemistry, felt that something had to be the matter with a man in his thirties if his sex drive was as low as Mark's.

"It's like pulling teeth," she complained. "I don't get it. We used to be so in love. Now it feels like I have to tiptoe around him to even get a good-night kiss. And I feel so ugly." Her eyes welled with tears. "There's got to be something wrong because he doesn't seem to want me anymore."

"I do want you. There's nothing wrong with you and nothing wrong with our relationship," he retorted. "It's just that I have so much on my mind these days." Mark, a newly appointed university professor, went on to grumble about his career. "There are lots of pressures at work," he explained. "I have all these deadlines for publication coming up, I'm serving on far too many committees, and my students are putting a lot of demands on my time right now." He paused and then added, "Having sex with Sheila feels like just another demand. I love her and I love our time together, but I am just too stressed."

But Sheila didn't believe it. She doubted his sincerity and worried that their relationship was falling apart. Their lack of intimacy increased her doubts about her own attractiveness and made her feel more depressed. But in trying to figure out what was wrong, they had ignored the most important piece of the puzzle: their struggle with infertility. They had been trying to conceive for eighteen months.

After identifying that infertility was, in fact, at the root of their problems, it became clear that Mark was feeling pressure not only at work, but also in his ability to perform sexually. He finally admitted: "You know, there are times when I'd actually like to have sex, but I'm afraid we'll use up the good sperm, if there even are any."

What Does it Mean to be a Man or a Woman?
The Loss of Sexual Identity

Mark's last comment, "If there even are any," almost thrown out as an aside, was key to understanding his underlying insecurity and self-blame. *"This is my fault!"* was being silently shouted throughout the room. Mark unconsciously believed that if Sheila wasn't pregnant, he was doing something wrong. His efforts to reassure Sheila that there was nothing wrong with *her* reinforced his conviction that *he* was to blame. "After all," he explained, "someone has to be." Rather than make an effort sexually, and have his "failure" thrown in his face month after month, Mark, without realizing it, was choosing to avoid the situation altogether. Although they had yet to see an infertility specialist and begin any testing, his assumption that he was the cause of their reproductive trauma dictated his behavior—not just his avoidance of sex, but his role at the university as well. His desire for perfection and success at work was driven, in part, by his need to prove himself and his manliness.

Different from sexual intimacy, which is about the relationship between an individual and his or her partner, sexual identity has to do with how people feel about themselves as sexual beings. Infertility has a major impact on how we think about ourselves as men and women—and what it means to be masculine or feminine. Are you less of a man or woman if you can't have a child? The real answer, of course, is no, but it may feel like yes.

Sometimes in order to counteract these feelings, people try to prove their virility or femininity in other ways. Men, for example, may increase their sports activities—instead of jogging two miles a few times a week, there may be a sudden desire to train for a triathlon. Women may boost themselves by going on a shopping spree or trying to lose weight. In general, we've noticed that men tend to become more active to counter their loss of virility, while women more often retreat into depression.

These feelings of sexual inadequacy may lead people into fantasies of having extramarital relationships, which, if acted upon, are obviously destructive for the couple. Carl, a software engineer, found himself in a quandary because of his attraction to someone he worked with. "I have been feeling so unappealing lately that this flirtation with my co-worker has been wonderful. I fantasize about her and what it would be like," Carl said. "I don't want to jeopardize my marriage, but in the back of my mind I can't help but wonder if this other woman and I *would* be able to make babies."

It is often difficult for people to admit to these kinds of thoughts; they feel extremely guilty even though they haven't acted on their feelings. We let clients like Carl know that it is normal to feel these things, and very helpful to talk about them—but best in individual sessions with a therapist, rather than directly with their partner or in couples' sessions. Bringing these fantasies out into the open and talking about the feelings with a therapist helps you to understand rather than act on them. Please remember that it may well be the losses connected with infertility, rather than something wrong with your relationship, that drive the desire to look elsewhere.

Having a child feels like a proof to the world that you are a viable sexual being. The truth, however, is that you are just as much a woman or a man regardless of whether you have a child or not. It's the *feeling* that you are sexually diminished that needs to be addressed. Infertility can undermine your confidence in so many areas of your life that it's important to look for the possible connection whenever you feel insecure.

Is Nothing Sacred? The Loss of Sexual Privacy

When you decide to consult with an infertility specialist, you open yourself up to even more strains on this most intimate part of your life. Sex, which has already caused so much anxiety, feels even more labored with medical interventions. You are now faced with giving intimate details of your sexual activity to doctors, nurses, medical technicians, and hospital staff. What was once the most personal and private of acts now becomes clinical data for the medical staff to analyze. All sense of sexual privacy is lost. The act of making a child, which should have taken place in the comfort of your bedroom with the lights dimmed and soft music playing, now occurs in the sterile environment of a hospital or doctor's office under the glare of fluorescent lights and the clanging sounds of stainless steel instruments.

One way to get through this intrusion into your privacy is to embrace the bizarreness of it all. Using humor can be a great way to cut through the tense moments. "You have to know my mother-in-law to really appreciate this," Maxine began. "She is so prim and proper, and conservative beyond belief. One time we went to a movie together which had a pretty racy sex scene and she was shocked. She said, 'Why in heaven's name do they need to show that?' Anyway, Aaron and I took her out to dinner at her favorite restaurant the other night and out of the blue she said, 'You know, children (she always calls us children!), the way to get pregnant is for the woman to be on top. That's how we had you, Aaron dear.'"

"We were dumbfounded. Aaron started squirming and said, 'Yeah, right Mom' and I just looked down at my food hoping no one else in the restaurant heard her. At first I was angry. We have been to three specialists now; how dare she butt in that way and think that she knows more than they do? But later when we got home, we laughed our heads off. She just wants to help and maybe she did; we needed a good laugh."

Maxine and Aaron were able to put his mother's comments into perspective, but it is not always easy to do that. When it feels as if everybody else knows everything about your sex life, and has answers for you as well, you may need to remind yourself that making a baby is only one aspect of your sexual relationship. Nothing can take away the private closeness that you and your partner share.

When going through infertility treatment, not only must you cope with the embarrassment and loss of privacy in the doctor's office, you must also contend with your family and friends. Sometimes the people close to us know so many details about our treatment that their support begins to feel intrusive. They may ask when our next treatment is scheduled, how many eggs we produced, and if it worked this time around.

It can be especially difficult because couples often differ in their comfort level with sharing their situation with others. Karen and Joe had been struggling with infertility for three years but had told no one. By nature, Joe, an extremely private person, was raised to believe that "we don't air our dirty laundry. We keep our problems to ourselves." Karen, on the other hand, came from a close-knit family and was desperate to turn to her mother and sisters for support, as well as to her good friends. But she had kept their infertility secret at Joe's insistence. By the time they came in for help, Karen was not only overwhelmed with accumulated pain, anxiety, and stress, but she was furious with Joe for the control he exerted over her.

During therapy, it emerged not only that Joe was very private, but that their infertility was due to low sperm motility, of which Joe was deeply ashamed. By understanding the meaning that their infertility had for each of them, Joe and Karen could find a compromise. He became more comfortable with her talking to her closest family and friends, and she agreed not to talk about it with anyone else unless she checked with him first.

In chapter 9, we go into more detail on how to cope with the pressures imposed on us by the outside world, but what is essential to understand here is that you need to be aware, not only of your own needs for privacy, but of your partner's as well. We help our clients compromise with each other rather than get into power struggles about who is right or wrong. In fact, there really is no right or wrong way to handle these situations; the degree of privacy needed varies from person to person, and from moment to moment in the course of infertility treatment.

The Loss of Our Sense of Self

The accumulation of all these losses—those that are obvious as well as those that are less apparent—can shatter your sense of self and leave you feeling empty. The pieces of the puzzle that make up your identity have been scattered, damaged, and lost in the grueling course of infertility and its treatment.

Think back to Mary, when she removed her own clothing and donned a hospital gown for her laparoscopy. She felt anxious because of the upcoming surgery, but she was equally upset about losing a part of her identity—her sense of self as healthy and normal. The reality of being in a hospital setting for a diagnostic test disallowed denial. She was forced to replace one piece of the puzzle—I am healthy—with another—I am an infertility patient.

Leslie, the kindergarten teacher who was losing control over her class, also lost a fundamental piece of her identity. Having always taken pride in her teaching ability, Leslie was experiencing so much distress from her infertility that her sense of competence as a teacher was undermined. Feeling less competent at work, combined with not being able to have a baby, created a downward spiral of emotions that left her feeling depressed and inadequate.

Likewise, Mark's conflicts about sex made him feel less masculine. He struggled with sex not because he lacked desire for his wife, Sheila, but because his sense of self was challenged. Since Mark's idea of manliness was reduced to the act of insemination, then he was not doing his job. Because Sheila was not yet pregnant, he assumed it was his fault. His doubt that he could produce any good sperm revealed his low estimation of his abilities as a man; the shame he felt was due to this larger sense that his whole self, as he had defined it, was crumbling.

When you take on the identity of infertility patient, you are forced to define yourself differently. You no longer feel that you can rely on yourself; you have lost not only self-esteem, but also the sense of your own competence. You are in pieces rather than whole—as if someone has kicked the table on which your jigsaw puzzle is resting. You become consumed with trying to regain cohesion, so you can recognize yourself again. You may feel that the only way to accomplish this is to have a child. That's what makes us feel so desperate.

In chapter 5, we explore in more depth *why* our identity is so traumatized by infertility. Understanding why we are shaken to the core gives us a plan for putting the pieces of the puzzle back together again, and thus helps us heal.

Acknowledging the Losses

The first step in healing from the multiple losses of infertility is to acknowledge that they exist; only then can they be mourned. As we have suggested throughout this chapter, bringing the losses out into the open and talking about them—with your partner, a support group, a therapist, or even talking to yourself or writing in your infertility diary—is the best way of gaining control over them. We have found with our clients that hiding from the losses creates more problems; trying to deny them causes more distress. Only by recognizing the powerful impact that these multiple losses have on us can we take the second step toward healing— which is to learn to grieve them.

Four

How Can I Be an Adult if I Don't Become a Parent?

James and I come from large families," Gretchen began. "I have five brothers and sisters, he has three, and we all live fairly close by. Whenever there's a family get-together—at least once a month with all their kids' birthdays and holidays—we go to their houses; they never come to ours. Whenever we invite them over, they say, 'Why don't you come here instead? It's easier for us; the kids have all their stuff here.' I understand that it's more convenient for us to go to them, but it makes me angry—like they're the grown-ups and we're not."

Out of all their siblings, James and Gretchen are the only ones without children; they have wrestled with infertility for over three years. With each family gathering, they feel more and more like outsiders. "Even though neither of us is the youngest, when we get together it *feels* that way," Gretchen continued. "It feels like James and I should be sitting at the kids' table."

What Gretchen describes, as do so many of our clients, is the regressive pull of infertility. It's startling to hear accomplished and successful men and women talk about themselves in child-like terms: feeling lost, helpless, or stuck. And these sentiments may hit harder at times when you feel particularly vulnerable—when you've had a failed cycle, when a co-worker goes on maternity leave, when someone asks the dreaded question about having kids.

You may not be consciously aware of this underlying "somehow I'm not an adult yet if I haven't had a child" thought. But we find that the loss of confidence and autonomy that comes with adulthood permeates the stories that our clients share with us.

Why does infertility makes you feel like a child? What is it about the experience that makes successful people in their twenties, thirties, and early forties question their status as adults in the adult world? What does infertility do to the deep inner workings of our psyches to derail us from feeling as though we really do belong at the "grown-up table"?

We know that growing up isn't magically completed when you turn twenty-one. Nor does it suddenly cease when you start your first job, move away from home, or get married. While our bodies stop growing during adolescence, our psyches continue to develop throughout our life span. Psychological maturation is a lifelong process, and adulthood is marked by specific developmental phases, just like childhood and adolescence. The milestones of adulthood that are thwarted by infertility are perhaps the most hidden losses of all, and may well cause the most distress.

The developmental processes that underlie true psychological maturity include:

- separating from your own parents: developing a psychological independence from your parents
- strengthening your adult identity: gaining confidence in yourself as you increase responsibility in your life
- forming intimate relationships: from finding someone to share a life with to starting a family of your own
- giving to a future generation: fulfilling a need to leave something for the future

Although there are many ways to achieve these milestones successfully, parenthood can and does play a key role. That's why you may be at the top of your profession, but shrivel up inside when someone asks if you have kids. You may feel as if you have finally worked through all your "stuff" with your mother until she tries to comfort you following an infertility procedure, or worse, laments that you have not given her a grandchild. It's important to recognize that infertility is not only an individual and marital crisis—it is a developmental crisis as well.

So we are left with the question: how can you be an adult if you can't be a parent? You can begin by uncovering and acknowledging how your hope of becoming a parent—your realization of your own *parental identity*—is one way in which we come to see ourselves as grown.

Becoming Your Own Person

"When I was a little girl, people would always ask, 'What do you want to be when you grow up?' Sometimes I wanted to be a doctor, sometimes a fireman, sometimes a teacher. But always, I wanted to be a mom. My mom had five kids by the time she was thirty. And here I am, almost forty, and not even close to being a mom," said Sandy, diagnosed with polycystic ovaries. "To me, that's what being a grown-up was really all about."

Why does Sandy, a family-law attorney, feel so unfulfilled, even though to others she's an extremely competent and successful adult? First, regardless of your age or circumstances, parenthood entails the passing of the generational torch—you are now the parent, and someone else is the child. But as Sandy so painfully expressed, becoming a parent does even more than that. It helps us consolidate our identities as separate from our parents—now we get to be the ones making the rules instead of the child always following them.

Becoming emotionally and physically independent, and maturing into an individual who is psychologically autonomous from one's parents, is a process that changes and varies throughout life. Psychologists refer to this developmental task as separation—the the process by which we become our own person with an identity separate from our parents. Separation does not mean a severance of ties; rather, the goal is to reconnect to those close to us in new and different ways, once you've developed your own identity. As Max, 30, remarked, "Now that I'm married, I relate to my dad differently. Like we are friends, with similar lifestyles, rather than as father and boy."

Feeling like a Child Again

The life event of infertility can make us especially vulnerable to the regressive pulls of childhood. "Whenever we visit my folks," Connie said, "Chip and I stay in my old bedroom. It hasn't changed since I left home and it makes me feel little—like I'm not in charge—like I'm a kid again. I used to feel it before we were trying to have our own family, but now it's really bad." With infertility, your sense of autonomy may feel precarious. Even if you have achieved professional goals and have not been dependent on your family for years, you may suddenly feel insecure and inadequate. You may turn to parents for financial help, undermining your sense of providing for yourself. At times, your family's support may come as a welcome relief; it can feel good to let someone take care of you for a while. But at other times, you may feel as if you are going backward. Rather than feeling adult and self-reliant, you feel childlike, needy, and out of control.

Conflicts about dependency can affect the potential grandparents as well as the infertile couple. Your parents, used to you as independent, may feel awkward and unsure of how to help. They may want to help financially with the exorbitant costs of infertility treatment, but such an offer may feel like a burden as well as a relief. Joan, 38, was torn about asking her parents for money for her first IVF cycle. "When we were remodeling the kitchen in our house," she said, "my parents offered to help. They went to a kitchen store with us and began talking to the salesman as if it were their kitchen! It made me so angry, like I was a little kid and invisible. I'm worried the same thing will happen now; that if they help us out financially, they will become overly involved in my treatment. And yet, if they don't help out, we won't be able to afford this." Feeling trapped by the financial costs, Joan was battling the regressive pull of dependency on her parents.

Growing Up Is Hard to Do

The separation process is especially important to the reproductive story at three important developmental stages. The first occurs in early childhood, during the toddler and preschool years, when we first begin to form ideas and expectations about what it means to be a person in our own right, and then make the transition from the intense, one-to-one attachments to our parents into the social world of school. The second happens during adolescence, when we begin to explore our sexuality and form more mature attachments to people outside of our immediate family. The third takes place in early adulthood, and is often focused on the transition to parenthood.

It's important to recognize that the passage through each phase does not mean that separation is complete. Just as physical growth occurs in spurts, so does separation. Moving through one phase marks a readiness to move on to the next. Each phase helps us become more of our own person, and foreshadows the realization of our autonomy, as well as our ability to establish intimate relationships with others as adults.

Yet the helplessness and loss of control that infertility evokes reawakens feelings from early childhood. What should be effortless, what everyone else seemingly can do with ease, is not happening for you. You may feel the same frustration as the toddler when you can't do it yourself. The grown-up world that you envisioned when you were young may feel out of reach when your reproductive story doesn't go as you had imagined it would. Your growing up feels thwarted, just as it did in childhood when your parent told you: "No, you're not big enough yet."

In turn, the shame and embarrassment that often accompany

infertility, when intimate details of your feelings and your sexuality feel all too public, can remind you of similar feelings from your adolescence, when the need for sexual and emotional privacy and independence was paramount. And like an adolescent, no longer a child but still not part of the world of grown-ups, you may feel as if you will be stuck at thirteen forever.

Feeling Stuck

The third phase of the separation process often focuses on the transition to parenthood. If infertility is interfering with this developmental stage, you may be faced with a painful question: how can you feel like a full adult if you are unable to become a parent?

There are no easy answers, but we find that when you understand the separation issues you might be struggling with unconsciously, and the role that parenthood can play as you mature into adulthood, this limbo can be easier to bear.

Becoming Equals

Having a child allows you to connect with your parents adult-to-adult, rather than as child-to-parent. Without infertility or other reproductive traumas, having a child means you can get to know your parents in a different way, as you learn what it's like to be a parent yourself. "Once I became a parent, I felt like I understood my own parents so much better," said Claudia, 38. "My mother always worried about me. Her constant concern drove me crazy; I wanted to be left alone. I remember her saying, 'Just wait until you have kids of your own. You'll see.' And she was right! Now I worry just as much."

But it is more difficult to feel identified with or "equal" to your parents, if you can't be a parent yourself. Again, you may not consciously be aware of this; it was only after Claudia had children that she understood the connection. What helps is to heighten your awareness of what might be occurring internally, so you can better cope with the strain.

Cassie described the subtle shift she felt whenever she and her mother and sister got together. "My mother and sister, who has a two-year-old, have a connection with each other that I don't. At first I thought I was jealous of my sister. We used to compete a lot as teenagers. She's three years older, and in high school she had such cool friends. Back then I was so envious of her. And then I thought maybe it's because my sister needed advice about my niece and she would only listen to my mother. I guess I'm still envious. But it's more than that. There's this feeling I have that they are both adults and I'm not."

Cassie still struggles with her feelings about this difference, but knowing what's going on makes her feel more in control when she's with her family. Identifying what's lurking beneath the surface won't make the feelings go away, but you'll be better able to handle what you do feel.

My Parents Had Kids, Why Can't I?

Competition between siblings, as with Cassie and her sister, is readily understandable. Less obvious are the competitive feelings you may have with your parents—after all, they were able to have children, so why can't you? Feeling like an equal with a parent involves resolving the natural (and normal) sense of competition we feel with them. Consciously or not, we want their approval and their admiration, and often we want to show by our achievements that we are just as good at things as they are—if not better.

Again, having a child of your own helps you achieve a sense of equal footing with your parents. If you struggle with infertility, however, you can't quite resolve the competitiveness. Infertility prevents you from sharing the title of "parent" along with your own parents.

The intergenerational impact of this loss may be profound, affecting not only you but your parents as well. June, 62, the mother of four, was distressed that she and her daughter Amy, 34, were no longer close. Amy had been trying to get pregnant for over two years. "I only know they were trying because at the beginning she would confide in me," June said sadly.

June was hurt by Amy's growing distance and didn't understand Amy's need to flaunt her material successes. "This isn't like her," June said. "She talks about how much money she has, and how much more cultured she is than me. Even when I try to be supportive, she rebuffs me, like I'm not good enough for her." When June understood that her daughter's infertility made Amy feel inadequate, especially in light of June's own fertility, she could empathize with her daughter. June also recognized her own dreams of being a grandparent, and how sad she was that this was not happening as planned. As June got in touch with her own grief, she understood the depth of her daughter's trauma. She came to see that Amy's put-downs were Amy's way of competing in an arena other than parenthood. Amy was struggling to feel like a successful adult, even at her mother's expense.

The more you can recognize and understand these normal feel-

ings of competition, the less distress you will feel. Talking about
your struggles with your parents can also help reduce this sense of
competition.

By doing so, you may discover more about your parents' reproductive stories and find out that your parents also experienced reproductive traumas. It is sad, but true, that events like miscarriages
and infertility are often not discussed, even within one's own family. Linda, 34, has a brother fourteen years older. Only when she
confided in her mother about her own infertility did Linda learn
that her mother had three miscarriages in the years after her
brother's birth and didn't expect to become pregnant again. She
was thrilled when she finally conceived Linda. Thanks to their
conversation, Linda's mother could support and empathize with
Linda, which she had not expected.

Your parents' experience may also influence you in ways you
didn't realize. When Jason talked with his mother, she revealed
that she experienced several miscarriages before his birth. Then,
when Jason was three years old, his younger twin brothers were
born prematurely. "I remember being confused when my brothers
were born," Jason said. "I had to stay with my neighbors until my
grandparents arrived. At first it was okay, even fun, but I missed
my mother. I thought maybe my parents were never going to be
home to take care of me again. I really didn't understand what was
happening."

As an adult, Jason was so terrified of having multiples, and going through what his parents had experienced, that he was unwill-
ing to pursue infertility treatment. Understanding how his parents'
trauma made him so resistant to medical intervention finally freed
him to reconsider using it.

As you uncover and articulate your reproductive story, it can help to learn more, if possible, about your parents' stories. Many of our clients have found it eases their own burdens if they open up to their parents, and sometimes they have learned surprising things about their family history. Even a small exchange of information can help you see yourself differently in relation to your parents.

Of course, it's easy for us to say, "Talk to your parents about this." We know how difficult it can be to discuss something as private as your struggles to have a baby. It runs counter to the autonomy you have worked so hard to attain, and the privacy of your sexual life. You may want to protect yourself from their disappointment at not becoming grandparents, because you already feel guilty and sad. Or you may not feel comfortable accepting financial help from them. You may also worry that your parents may seem pushy or insensitive in their own discomfort and sense of helplessness about your situation.

So consider what's right for you as you decide whether or not to have these conversations with your parents. If you feel strongly that you don't want to do so, take that as a sign that you aren't ready to talk yet, so there's no need to force a conversation. If you do go ahead, try to anticipate how you and they might respond. Always know that if the conversation takes a negative turn, you can be prepared to end it by simply stating that you have talked enough for now, that you appreciate their concern (give them the benefit of the doubt), and that you can talk more later. This gives everyone time to digest what has transpired and rethink his or her responses.

Reworking Old Conflicts

Having your own family also gives you the opportunity to work through conflicts from your past. Making decisions about how you want to raise your children is another way to separate from your parents and become an individual in your own right. For example, if your parents were distant or unavailable, you may plan to be more nurturing and engaged with your child. Not only does this allow you to heal old wounds, you can also pass on lessons learned from your parents' errors and not repeat their mistakes. (Of course you'll make some of your own!)

Infertility deprives us of the chance to repair old damage to our sense of self, and to prove we can be different from—and in some ways better than—our own parents. This happened to Carly, from chapter 2, who had a troubled relationship with her parents. Her parents were still teenagers when she was born, leading to a chaotic and troubled family situation. Consequently, she and her husband, Vince, waited until they were older and financially secure before trying to start a family. "I thought I was fixing things in a way so that my kids wouldn't grow up with the same kind of stress," she said. "But now, even though I planned it so well, I can't have a family the way I thought I would."

Not only does having a family give you a chance to rework the negative, you can also pass on the positive. As Laura, who reminisced in chapter 2 about how her mother made doll clothes for her "babies," said, "My mom also made the best oatmeal cookies! I have the recipe and can't wait to bake for my own kids. The things I remember loving I want to do for my children as well."

How Can You Achieve "Separation" if You Don't Have a Baby?

It seems so unfair to lose these opportunities to continue your development as an adult. Haven't you already lost too much?

Again, we don't mean to suggest that you are not adult if you don't have children. (Many people have children and still don't achieve autonomy from their parents; many others without children find other satisfying ways to do so.) You have likely separated from your parents in many significant ways: in your career, your relationships, your friendships, and your finances. But when you want to have a child, and cannot, it sometimes feels as though you are not quite the same as—not quite on par with—all the other adults who are parents. If you want to become a parent, infertility interrupts your sense of completion and accomplishment, no matter what else you have done.

Recognizing these feelings as part of the infertility experience is an important step in overcoming them. You feel traumatized not only by the fact of infertility, but also by the delay in completing this developmental task.

It can help, though, to think of other ways to accomplish this goal, or consider ways that you've already done so. How else do you feel separate and independent from your parents, and like an adult in your own right? How are you glad to be different from your parents, or proud to be similar, that don't have to do with having children? Are there other people in your life who see you as a competent adult? Ask yourself these kinds of questions, and periodically remind yourself of the answers.

Consolidating Your Adult Identity:
Who Am I if I Can't Have a Baby?

As you mature into adulthood, you consolidate an internal sense of who you are. The jigsaw puzzle pieces that make up the self fit together in new ways as you gain new responsibilities. Getting married, moving into one's own home, receiving a promotion at work, or having a child are all ways in which the course of adult development moves forward and strengthens your sense of self.

When you decide to have a baby, your identity shifts from being the child to being the parent, from being a couple to being a threesome, from being a husband and wife to being a father and mother. And as with any life transition, you must let down your guard to make room for your new identity, just as you did in adolescence when you shifted from child to adult. Just as a woman's pelvis loosens and widens to make room for the fetus, so our psychological structures loosen to attach to an infant and take on a parental identity. This often leaves us feeling extra vulnerable and emotional; we are excited, scared, confident, and nervous all at the same time. During this transition, we need to get to know our new selves, internally, just as we get to know a new neighborhood when we move.

If all goes well, and you conceive as planned, your psyche reconsolidates and progresses into the new identity—that of pregnant person/couple. You use the time of pregnancy to become gradually accustomed to this change. However, if you experience infertility at this point, the ground isn't merely shaky; it's like living through an earthquake. You feel as if you no longer know who you are; you feel confused and unbalanced. The psychological space you made to include a baby is empty. The lullabies in your mind are not being sung. The pieces of the puzzle don't seem to fit together anymore—all because infertility makes you lose sight of the whole picture. Rather than feeling that your identity is consolidating, you feel as if you are floundering.

"I'm falling apart at the seams," said Sarah, 29, with undiagnosed infertility. "I'm not able to concentrate and get frazzled when I try to make plans. I constantly doubt myself and my abilities. I just don't know who I am anymore."

Katherine, 36, also feels at a crossroads. Two years ago she quit her sales rep job, because she wasn't sure she wanted a career that required constant traveling. At first, the relief of not working was exhilarating. "I had so much free time, it felt like I was on vacation. I caught up with old friends and completed house projects that I'd been trying to get to for a long time. I was sure I would get pregnant quickly and everything would fall into place accordingly," she said.

Now she doesn't know what to do after two years of trying. Returning to work, in her mind, means giving up the idea of having a family. But she doesn't want to think of herself as a full-time infertility patient.

And Jenny, a chiropractor, is like many of our clients who tend to put their life on hold as they battle infertility. "I really want to open up my own practice," she said. "I keep waiting to get pregnant, and when I don't I get more frustrated that I haven't done this yet." When Jenny recognized what a hold her infertility had over her, she could move forward to fulfill the important "work" part of herself.

When you, like so many others, yearn for a label of "mommy"

or "daddy" that isn't forthcoming, you need to mourn this loss of your longed-for new identity. The trauma of infertility can be so overwhelming that it can take over and color how you feel about your entire adult self. We tell our clients to remember that your identity is not a single element, but a composite of the many different aspects of yourself. Being a parent, although a major piece of your adult sense of self, is still just one piece. It can bring relief to celebrate that your identity is made up of many different parts—not just the "having a baby" part. Keeping in mind all your parts—even making a list—helps you maintain perspective on this identity crisis, so you can feel strong as a person once again.

Longing for Connection: My Arms Ache to Hold a Baby

If growing up means being separate, adulthood can indeed loom as lonely and disconnected. The wish to regain a sense of connection with others is part of what motivates us to fall in love and have a family. When we find our partner, we may feel that we've found another part of ourselves. While the motivations for wanting children are varied and complex, one common result of this intimate connection with a partner is the wish to make a family together and build on the closeness you cherish and love. What better joy than to create something—a family—together.

Creating a family—whether it is having your own biological child, using donor technology, or adopting—has the potential to bond you and your partner in a new way. And whether you are a couple or a single parent, having a child sparks another very different intimate connection with another person—the relationship with your baby is unlike any relationship you have ever had before.

We long for the joy being a parent can bring. Corinne described this. "I watched as my friend's two-year-old ran to her and climbed into her lap. He snuggled into her arms and it was like the rest of the world was shut out. That's what I miss, that's what I want, that's why my arms ache as they do."

When you are going through infertility, you may feel that longing for your own family to such a degree that nothing else can satisfy it. There is no replacement; the baby you yearn for, to sing to, to love, and to nurture, is painfully absent. No magic words of advice can get rid of this pain. Sometimes there is nothing we can do but cry. These deep losses need to be grieved, which we discuss in chapter 8. Being aware that your longing—your unsung lullaby—is part of normal adult development may help you understand the depth of the despair you feel.

Giving to the Future

Another goal of adult development concerns our wish to leave something of ourselves for future generations. Psychologists call this the need for "generativity": how we ensure that not only our genes, but also our principles and values, will be passed along to generations to come. By giving to the future, we also give back to society and add meaning to our present lives. It's as if we've been students, absorbing life's lessons, and now we can teach the next generation. By doing so, we come to terms with our own mortality, knowing that we will, in some form, live on in others. Giving to the next generation can involve mentoring younger workers in your job, working on a cure for cancer, or like Laura, sharing a well-loved recipe.

Clearly, having a child is one of the most tangible ways to fulfill this need. Our family line continues, linking the past and future.

As Alice, 70, said, "Becoming a grandparent was one of the most thrilling experiences of my life. It felt as if I had finally come full circle, that I could see into my future. I hadn't been as aware of my own mortality when I had my kids, but now I can see how we pass the torch from one generation to the next. To see my son holding his baby—I cried."

Yet many of us feel frustrated like Rosa, a journalist and writer, infertile for four years with no clear diagnosis. She no longer feels that her work is an ideal way to give back. "Everything I attempt to do these days seems pointless. I used to feel so good when I knew someone was reading an article I had written, that somehow I was changing their life," she said. "But it has no meaning for me anymore. What I really want is to give to a child, *my* child, not just anyone who cares to read what I have written."

What happens when you are unable to have a biological child? Does this mean that you are unable to leave part of yourself for the future? For some couples, having a biological child feels like the only choice possible; they feel they must continue their genetic line. Other couples believe that raising a child and imparting their skills and values fulfills their wishes to give to the future, even if the child is not genetically connected to them. Those who remain childfree find other ways to fulfill their generative needs.

Each person and couple must come to terms with their wish to give to the future. The problem arises when infertility interferes with your particular reproductive story, when it feels as if everything—not just your becoming a parent—has been thrown off course. If your greatest wish is to leave a biological child for the future, and you are faced with the prospect of being unable to do so, the other ways you express your generativity and contribute to the future may feel like pale substitutions for what you really long for. Only by understanding the developmental needs you are trying to meet, and facing the losses and changes in your own reproductive story, can you regain at least partial satisfaction in what you are already doing to give to the future.

Maybe you'll give back through your business contributions, your artistic creations, or your volunteer work. Margaret decided to make quilts for her nieces and nephews. "A piece of me goes into every quilt," she said. "It makes me feel great to think they may even pass these quilts to their own children."

When you step back, even a little bit, from the struggles of infertility and think about how you contribute to the world, you can discover sources of satisfaction that will be there throughout your life. So we suggest these three steps. First, reflect on what you have to offer. That's a lot! Second, please continue doing these things while you are undergoing infertility treatment. Finally, recognize that these contributions are important sources of meaning in your life that will continue regardless of the outcome of your next cycle.

How you choose to give to the future is up to you. What's important is regaining pride in what you have to offer.

How Can I Be an Adult If I Can't Have a Baby?

When we consider the complexity of growing up, and what may be accomplished psychologically by having a child, we can appreciate how deeply we are touched by the trauma of infertility. Although there are many ways to achieve adult milestones and fulfill our adult needs for autonomy, growth, intimacy, and continuity, having a baby can be a particularly meaningful one.

Can you be an adult if you don't have a baby? Of course, but when you long for a baby, it is difficult to imagine anything else that will fulfill the adult needs covered in this chapter. Indeed, as we have seen with so many people we have worked with, the numerous ways that people *do* accomplish these tasks often get discounted when infertility becomes part of the picture. Prior to infertility, you may have felt proud of and satisfied with your relationships with your partner and friends, your professional accomplishments, your home, and your life. But all this seems to pale in the face of infertility.

Getting thrown off course of achieving these developmental milestones by infertility is an enormous loss. Again, it is a loss of opportunity, and, because the needs are most often unconscious, and unfold quite naturally when all goes well, we may feel even more helpless and bewildered by our diminished self-esteem or the loss of meaning in our life due to infertility. By becoming aware of how infertility derails these normal and necessary tasks of adulthood, you will be able to develop other ways of meeting these goals. You can be conscientious in setting clear boundaries with your parents, maintaining close relationships, recognizing your value as a person, and contributing to society. By remembering that parenthood does not define adulthood, and that infertility does not define you as a person, you will be able to continue your growth as a person throughout this ordeal.

Five

If Everyone Else Can Do This, Why Can't I?

Like a left hook coming out of nowhere, infertility delivers a powerful punch right at your core. You are failing at something that seems so easy for everyone else. You may feel out of synch with your peers, your family, even society at large. You may feel so awful that you want to hide in shame.

The loss of self-esteem and confidence that comes with infertility can be truly overwhelming. The negative thoughts you may harbor about yourself hurt terribly. And it's hard to fight back when you feel knocked down and depleted.

"I feel beat up," Marsha began. At thirty-four, Marsha has undergone multiple surgeries for endometriosis, yet her prognosis remains poor. "It's not just the surgeries that make me feel like I'm in the ring with Mike Tyson. It's the daily grind, that ever-present awareness that I'm different than most other women. It makes me feel like something is wrong with me, not just the physical part of me, but *all* of me."

In this chapter we look at several external and internal factors that can undermine your self-esteem, such as:

- the media's emphasis on how easy it is to get pregnant
- our family-oriented culture
- the narcissistic injury that you experience
- your personal suffering of the silent pain of infertility

We have found with our clients that the more they understand about themselves, the better they feel. Being able to pinpoint where and why negative feelings arise and how they can take hold of you lets you separate those feelings from the rest of who you are. Holding on to what is positive about yourself in the midst of feeling demoralized and defeated lets you get back in the ring again.

The Myths We Live by

Media Myths

Bridget, thirty-one years old and taking Clomid for the second time, was peeved. "It seems so easy for everyone else," she said. "My friends are popping out kids like crazy. And then you pick up *People* filled with glowing photos of all these celebrities—not only are they pregnant and happy, they're stunning! Their bodies are gorgeous, their hair is impeccable, their makeup is flawless . . . you name it, it's perfect! They make it seem so simple—so what's my problem?"

Celebrity pregnancies plaster the pages of fashion and parenting magazines, sending the message that everyone can (and should) be seven months pregnant and look dazzling, even in their forties! It's too easy to absorb this media message that pregnancy is an easy and natural state—and start agonizing, *"What's wrong with me? Why is my body not working right? Why can everyone do this except me?"*

What you rarely see are the stories of the great lengths that some women have to go to to get pregnant. Of course, celebrities are entitled to their privacy, but only a brave few have chosen to share publicly their struggles to get pregnant. Rarely do we hear anything negative about pregnancy in the media. We don't read about the miscarriages and we certainly don't read about infertility, even though one out of every six couples may be experiencing it. These troubles are not broadcast nearly as loudly, if at all.

Instead, the implied message is that having a baby is predictable and expected, within our control, and that, indeed, anyone can do it. The truth is that pregnancy is not a sure thing at all. How the pregnancy will go, and whether or not a woman will even become pregnant is unpredictable and out of anyone's control. The myth that getting pregnant is effortless is so deeply embedded in our collective culture that it comes as an enormous blow when it is not easy. In fact, for some of us, getting pregnant is the hardest thing we have ever tried to do.

Before you experienced infertility, before you even tried to conceive, you may have had some trepidation. We have found in our practice that some women will worry about gaining too much weight while pregnant, while others are concerned about miscarrying. Or they feel nervous about labor and delivery, or that something might be wrong with the baby. But people rarely worry about infertility until it happens. And when it does, it takes center stage in our lives. Not only are you not living up to the airbrushed images of becoming the ideal parent, you can't even audition for the part. It is not surprising that your self-esteem takes a nosedive when you can't live up to your own expectations, or what you believe to be society's expectations.

The Myths of Reproductive Technology

Advances in reproductive technology also contribute to the cultural myth that pregnancy is in our control. Although ART is far from perfect, it does give us a sense—perhaps a false one—that we will be assured of a successful outcome. Although ART has improved over the years, the chances of having a "high-tech" baby from non-donor eggs through IVF are still only about 25 percent for women under thirty-five; for older women the chances are even less, according to 2001 nationwide statistics compiled by the Centers for Disease Control. A disconnect exists between the *reality* of what ART can do and the *hope* it holds for so many of us. This is not to say that couples should avoid using assisted technology. Not at all. But be wary of the myth that the technological advances will *guarantee* you a baby—that's what becomes the trap for so many.

This was true for Nell and Patrick. Both are now thirty-eight, and have talked about having a baby for about ten years. "Having children was always something we wanted to do—eventually. But the time just never seemed right," Nell said. "Either I was in school, or Patrick was. First he got his MBA while I worked. Then it was my turn and I went back to school for my MBA. And then Patrick went to work for a start-up company and it was so time consuming we rarely had time for each other. I realized it was going to be harder after thirty-five, but it never bothered me because so many people use artificial means to have children. I just figured we would too."

Many women, like Nell, are aware that their biological clock is ticking, but still put off having children because they know they can utilize ART. Sometimes women we work with, who are still menstruating regularly, think that they are as fertile at thirty-five as they were at twenty-five. The reality is that at age thirty, your chance of conceiving is only 20 percent per month; by age forty, it drops to only 5 percent per month, according to the American Society for Reproductive Medicine (ASRM).* Another prevailing belief is that thanks to ART we can get pregnant without too much trouble. That's what the media says and that's usually the punchline of the stories our friends tell us. What's not told nearly as often are the stories of the couples for whom ART never worked.

And how can someone say ART isn't too much trouble? The toll that ART can take on people's psychological and financial state can be astronomically high. So why, in spite of not-so-favorable odds and the enormous cost to our emotions and pocketbooks, do we presume that ART will answer our prayers? It's because our desire to have children is so strong. We will go to great lengths to realize the dream of having a baby and fulfill our reproductive story in spite of the fact that ART can be so trying—physically, mentally, and economically.

Cultural Myths

Ours is a family-centered society. As we discussed in chapter 3, infertile couples lose a sense of fitting in—with peers, with their family, and with society at large. There is a tacit cultural expectation that married couples will have children. Couples who choose

*Age and Fertility: A Guide for Patients, 2003.

not to have children do not feel the same pressures as infertile couples, yet they too can feel out of the loop when it comes to cultural expectations. But those of us who have not consciously made the choice to be childfree, but have had the decision forced upon us, feel stuck in limbo—out of step with what we expect of ourselves as well as what others expect of us. All of these factors contribute to a diminished sense of well-being and sense of self.

Valerie, who has been married for eight years and has tried numerous medical interventions over the past six years, is hyperaware of not fitting the mold. Her sense of self gets battered with each passing month, and Mother's Day has become a symbolic marker of her personal failure. "For me, it's the worst," she said. "I invariably spend the day in bed. Of course I call my mom, but there is no way I can partake in my family's traditional get-together."

Like Valerie, women and men who can't have children feel sorely out of place. "Lately I've been wondering, what's the point of getting married if you can't have kids?" she asked. "It's not that I don't love my husband, but this isn't my idea of what a family is. I want to be able to celebrate Mother's Day—but as a mom."

Why Do I Feel So Bad?

We've explored above how external societal factors—such as the myth of the perfect pregnancy portrayed by the media, along with cultural demands and expectations—can contribute to the sense that you are not up to par. And while you feel attacked from the outside, it's likely that inside you're chipping away at your self-esteem as well. Infertility changes how you envision yourself and your future and can cause feelings of worthlessness and failure, shame and guilt. No wonder your self-esteem plummets.

Delores, who has been trying for three years, recently received her invitation to her twenty-year high school reunion. "I was excited when I first got the notice. I went to my ten-year and it was a blast," she said. "But then it came over me like a wave. How could I possibly show my face?" At her ten-year reunion, very few of her high school friends had children. "A lot of people weren't even married then, but now I'm sure the conversations will be about kids, how many, and what ages. I don't think I could stand it. What will everyone say about me?"

What was really bothering Delores, though, had nothing to do with what others might say. "You know, it's my own embarrassment that's upsetting me. It's my own feelings about *me*—I'm my own worst critic when it comes to not having children." When she identified and understood that she was the source of her feelings of shame—not others—she was able to bolster herself by monitoring and "turning off" her internal critic, and attend her reunion.

Why is it that infertility wreaks such havoc with how you feel about yourself? What are the psychological mechanisms at play? Having a better understanding of these internal emotional systems will help in dealing with the trauma of infertility.

Changes in Your Self
Career Shifts

When you decided to have a baby, you opened yourself up to a new and life-altering situation. Whether you are in a traditional marriage, in a gay or lesbian relationship, or have decided to become a single parent—no matter how you arrange it—becoming a parent means that you are dealing with new psychological issues and realities.

As discussed in chapter 4, as soon as you begin planning to have a baby, you start to modify the way you think about yourself and your partner. The twosome of the couple becomes a threesome as your sense of self incorporates parental responsibilities. Often couples literally need to "make room"—deciding to start a family often motivates a couple to move from a smaller home to a larger one or change neighborhoods to live closer to family or to be in a good school district.

Making room for a baby may also influence career decisions. Monica, who worked for several years as a hospital nurse, ran the cardiac intensive care unit before she decided to switch to a job as a school nurse. "Even though I took a major pay cut, and a less prestigious and stimulating job, I decided to make this change so that I could still work, but have a more flexible schedule," she said.

Hal, an engineer by training, was trying to make it as a musician. When he and his wife started talking about having a family, the idea instilled a new sense of responsibility. "I can't believe it," he chuckled. "Suddenly I became interested in investments and minivans!" His music career became an avocation as he took on a full-time position as an engineer. "I was excited at first—the money was great, we were building toward something, had something to look forward to. But now, it's all a bust."

Maybe like Hal and Monica, you've been willing to make a career change and modify your personal ambitions in order to satisfy your stronger desire to have a family. Had you been able to have children as you had planned, these career shifts would have seemed right. But now you are suffering a double loss: not only is your reproductive story not unfolding according to plan, you also need to readjust your feelings about the career choices you've made.

You may also find that infertility affects your career. Ginny, a certified public accountant, found that the daily ultrasounds necessary to monitor ovulation drastically cut into her workday, and she opted to take a leave of absence. "Not only was the treatment too disruptive, I just couldn't concentrate. But staying at home is no picnic either," she said. "With so much time on my hands, I can't help but think about getting pregnant all the time. To top it off, there seems to be an endless parade of baby strollers being pushed down my street during the day. I just can't win."

Identity Shifts

As we discussed in chapter 4, our parental identity begins prior to the birth of a baby; we become psychological parents well before we become biological ones. When Hal decided not to pursue music professionally, he was consciously thinking about financial security, but underlying that was the unconscious development of his identity as a father. As part of his reproductive story, he wanted to become a better provider for his family-to-be and live up to his ideal of what a father should be.

This identity shift puts you in a psychologically vulnerable state; you may wonder if you will be up to the task and be successful as a parent. You may feel unsure: can you fill your parents' shoes? Or you may wonder if you've made the right choices, in addition to feeling ambivalent about past decisions during this transition. Did you delay childbearing to pursue a career? Are you now struggling with age-related infertility? Now, after finally coming to the decision to start a family and making the necessary psychological and practical adjustments, what a blow you are experiencing when that hoped-for baby doesn't arrive.

The changes we go through in preparation for having a family are profound, and can leave people feeling vulnerable even when all goes according to plan. It's worth reiterating that the feelings we have about becoming a parent—both positive and negative—are all normal, occur whether we are consciously aware of these changes or not, and happen as soon as we think about having a baby. At this critical juncture, our hopes and dreams for the future, our feelings about our past, our perceptions about ourselves and our parents, and our achievement of the ongoing developmental tasks of adulthood all come together. And because this is such a vulnerable period, we are at much greater risk for wounds to our self-esteem.

Healthy Narcissism

If all goes well, and pregnancy and birth move forward without problems, you may sail through this critical juncture with only the normal psychological growing pains. If, however, your reproductive experience is traumatic, you're in for a psychological beating.

Psychologists use the term *narcissistic injury* to explain what happens to one's self-esteem when it suffers a blow, as it does when we undergo infertility. To clarify and define a few terms: while *narcissism* is often thought of negatively as excessive self-centeredness, grandiosity, and need for admiration, it has a positive dimension, which is an essential part of a vital and dynamic person. *Healthy narcissism* is defined as concern for the self. Looking inward, understanding your motives and feelings, and paying attention to your needs are all crucial in feeling whole and worthy. Solid self-esteem, a belief that you have something to offer, and self-confidence are all part of healthy narcissism, helping you to cope with the trials and tribulations of life. In other words, feeling good about yourself is not a bad thing.

Healthy narcissism develops unconsciously over the course of our lives. It grows from simple events like having others greet you with a smile when you are small, having a drawing praised and hung up for view on the refrigerator, doing well on an exam, hitting a home run, or getting complimented on a new hairstyle. Healthy narcissism is also built when you set a goal and meet it or master a challenging task.

Having a child is another way that people enhance their sense of positive narcissism. The pride people take in their children and their accomplishments reflects pride in themselves. Consider the saying "a chip off the ol' block"—it illustrates how parents feel when their children resemble them in looks or actions. Even when a couple has adopted or used donor technology, they are proud when their children take on their mannerisms and traits. A child can serve as a *narcissistic extension* of the self; in our offspring, we hope to see the best of ourselves.

It is natural to have expectations and hopes that our children will be similar to us and will be everything we want them to be— and more. Of course, it never turns out exactly that way; children develop and grow in their own ways, and in fact must do so eventually to separate from us, just as we had to separate from our own parents. It is also normal to fantasize about what our children might be like long before they are conceived. This is, in actuality, the essence of the reproductive story, and because we have thought about our children-to-be for so long, they may become idealized in our minds. The hope that our children will fulfill *our* longings is a normal part of the wish to have children.

It follows, then, that by not being able to have a child, we cannot extend ourselves through our children into the future. We are denied the fulfillment of watching them grow; we are denied the pride and delight of seeing their accomplishments as a reflection of our own achievement as a parent. A major part of us is missing, sad, and empty.

Having children may further enhance healthy narcissism by allowing people to undo—or redo—some of the painful events of their own childhood. If, for example, you were one of the last kids picked for the team, you can bet that as your own child approaches that age, you will remember your experience viscerally. Being able to revisit the feelings, but as an adult with an adult's perspective, brings new insight and understanding. Infertility denies us the opportunity to return to our own childhood and heal old wounds by becoming the parent we want to be.

Wounds to the Self

Rather than fueling your healthy narcissism, infertility causes a *narcissistic injury,* a feeling of damage to your sense of yourself as a whole person. Because the psyche is such an intangible concept, it can be hard to imagine what happens when it is injured, but like our bodies, you can think of the self as having an immune system. And like a virus attacking you, infertility attacks your "self-esteem immune system." Instead of feeling sick physically, you feel emotional pain. A narcissistic injury can make you feel like a failure, gravely undermining your healthy narcissism and your sense of being a fully functioning adult.

What Did I Do to Deserve This?

Healthy narcissism is further diminished by guilt. Time after time our clients come in feeling as if they are somehow to blame for their infertility. They blame themselves for not taking care of themselves well enough, for sexual encounters they may have had, or for birth control they may have used. Margot blames the IUD she used for many years. "My doctors reassured me that it didn't cause any problems, but I'm not convinced," she said. "They can't find anything else wrong. Of course I think it's my fault for using the IUD in the first place."

Women may also feel an enormous sense of regret, failure, and guilt if they have had an ectopic pregnancy, miscarriage, or other pregnancy loss. Irene, who has had three miscarriages in as many years, said: "I don't know why my babies are not surviving. No one has been able to figure it out. My womb, which I always thought of as being a safe haven, is apparently not. What is it about me that causes my babies to die? It's not their fault that I can't keep them, so it must be mine." By idealizing her womb and her babies, Irene is left with no choice but to blame herself. Yet she feels at fault for something she truly cannot control.

Men can experience this as well. Todd feels guilty about partying when he was younger. "In college, I did drugs, drank a lot with the guys, had lots of casual sex," he confessed. "At the time, I didn't think much about it. But maybe I don't deserve to be a father. Maybe I'm paying for my bad actions of the past." Todd's sperm motility problems may not be connected to his past partying ways, yet he psychologically needs to find a reason for his infertility, even if it outweighs logic.

We see too often that many women and men struggling with infertility find it more comforting to blame themselves than to have no answers at all. Many people gain a feeling of control over the situation if they can point to a reason for their infertility, even if the logic is faulty. They need to feel in control of something when it feels as though everything is going haywire. Feeling in control, even if it involves guilt, may actually feel better than having nothing to blame.

But take a closer look at this faulty logic. Feeling guilty only causes more pain to an already diminished sense of self. The next time you find yourself feeling guilty, stop and check in with yourself. What just happened to make you feel out of control? Does it really make you feel better to blame yourself? It never really helps to beat yourself up, especially for something that you have no power over. Once you see the pattern of your guilt and understand the reasons why you blame yourself for infertility, you can break this destructive cycle.

Unplanned Pregnancies, Abortions, and Guilt

Talking to our clients, we have found that those who have had an unplanned pregnancy in the past blame themselves the most for the infertility they are experiencing today. Infertility can heighten old feelings of guilt, remorse, and self-blame, whether the pregnancy was terminated or the child was given up for adoption. Women and men alike may be haunted by the questions: *Did I do the right thing? Was that my only chance?*

Abortion

Celeste, thirty-five-years-old and infertile for four years, had an unwanted pregnancy at age sixteen. Still a child herself, she knew she was too young to care for a child of her own. "Getting pregnant was a mistake and I admit to being irresponsible," she said. "My parents were horrified with me for getting pregnant, and supportive of my decision to have an abortion. My mom even came with me; I remember being very scared. Afterward, she arranged for me to have birth control. She said if I was going to have sex, do it responsibly. They really were great throughout the whole ordeal."

She added, "It's ironic, but because of that pregnancy, I always assumed that when I was ready, it would be easy to get pregnant again. I never thought there would be a problem."

Although Celeste had made the right decision for herself as a teenager, she questioned herself now that she so desperately wanted a child. "I feel very confused," she said. "I know I did the right thing back then. But a small part of me wonders if that was my only chance. I wonder if I am being punished. It's so weird to have these thoughts. . . . Knowing what I know now, though, I'm not sure what I would have done." Her voice trailed off. "You know," she continued, "if I wasn't having such difficulty having a baby now, this issue would be nonexistent. It's when you can't have something you want that you look for meaning wherever you can find it."

Having an abortion is clearly a very personal decision. Celeste had made the right choice for herself when she was faced with an unwanted pregnancy. She certainly wasn't thinking about infertility then. But when infertility becomes an issue later, it is common for many doubts about the decision to emerge.

Adoption

When a woman chooses to go through with a pregnancy and give her child up for adoption, she, too, may struggle with intense feelings of remorse and self-blame. And if, years later, she has problems getting pregnant when she wants to become a mother, the intensity of those feelings may return with a vengeance.

Beth decided to give up her son for adoption when she got pregnant at nineteen. "It was the best decision I could have made at that time," she said. "I knew I placed my son with good people, and it was right for me too. Raising a child at that time in my life—and as a single mother—would not have been a good thing." Beth was determined to finish college and establish a career.

Although Beth was comfortable with her decision at age nineteen, it was not without feelings of sadness and grief. "I was a basket case after Andrew was born. My emotions flip-flopped. One minute I was thrilled to be giving him to such great people, the next I wanted to touch him and hold him close. I didn't want to get attached to him, but somehow it happened anyway. I kept reminding myself to focus on the long-term. Even though I was feeling awfully sad, thinking about what would be best for the baby, and ultimately best for me, was what got me through it."

Ten years later, at the age of twenty-nine, Beth assumed that having been pregnant once, she would easily get pregnant again. So she was all the more shocked and stunned when she couldn't get pregnant right away. Her doctor discovered that an infection had left significant scar tissue in her uterus, greatly reducing her chances of conceiving. And with that news came an onslaught of feelings that she thought had been put to rest.

"After all these years, I feel like I am back in the delivery room. The actual birth was painful, of course, but not as painful as saying good-bye to Andrew. Now that I can't have a baby, I think maybe I shouldn't have gone through with the adoption. I know it's too late to change anything, but a hole in me has opened up once again," she said.

Like other of our clients who have given a baby up for adoption or have had an abortion, Beth felt like she had lost her only chance at parenthood; she blamed herself and felt like she was being punished for past decisions. Beth's reproductive story had veered off track not just once, but twice. The first time was at age nineteen. But at twenty-nine, when she most desired a child, and was ready psychologically and emotionally, her reproductive story again took a turn in an unforeseen direction. Her current reproductive trauma brought back powerful feelings of regret and remorse.

Celeste, Beth, and others who have had previous reproductive traumas need to grieve—or re-grieve—their prior losses, so they do not carry the added burden of guilt and sadness into their current crisis. (In chapter 8, we talk at length about how to grieve reproductive traumas.)

Silent Tears: The Shroud of Secrecy

"Whenever anyone asks me if I have children I don't know what to say," said Andrea. "I'm a private person; it's none of their business, but at the same time, I worry that they think I'm being rude for not answering their question . . . and selfish for not having kids. The truth is I am so ashamed, I can't tell."

This seemingly innocuous question—*"Do you have kids?"*—takes on new meaning when you are struggling to have a baby. Like Andrea, you may feel unsure of how to respond, and want to keep your infertility under wraps.

The need to conceal infertility and keep it private is yet another dimension of the trauma that affects the self. Because infertility is a narcissistic injury, we feel ashamed of it, ashamed of what we see as our failure. The damage we feel can fuel our withdrawal from others at the very time when we need support and nurturance. So many of the women and men we work with suffer a silent pain and sense of isolation. As noted in chapter 3, infertility can close us out of our circle of peers who are sharing the joys of new parenthood, so we often are uncomfortable talking about our issues. Feeling that no one could possibly understand, we retreat from others and keep our infertility a secret.

Hilary has been trying to have a baby for two years. At first, she thought about telling a few close friends that she was trying, but then when nothing happened, she decided to keep her travails private. Coming into therapy was a great relief; at last she could let some of her feelings out. She shared a recent work experience. "Everyone was gathered around, looking at pictures from a co-worker's baby shower. I felt so awful, so alone. I worry that if people at work know about my infertility, they won't treat me the same way—they wouldn't include me in sharing about their children because they would be afraid of hurting me," she said. "And I don't want people asking me about my treatment—it's private. I'm afraid I would be the fuel for office gossip."

"It's as if everybody is on one side of this fence, and I am on the other," she continued. "I can see through the gate, but I can't open it. It feels as if I will never, ever be the same as them; that's why I need to keep this a secret."

Like Hilary, the isolation is both felt by and created by people going through infertility. Sometimes it is intensified by your need to retreat from others in order to protect your fragile sense of self. But the damage to your sense of self adds to your need to withdraw, and consequently adds to your pain.

Sometimes, we are forced to reveal our fertility status when we would rather keep it private. Hilary was furious after a visit to a new dentist. "It took all I had to confide in him that I was trying to get pregnant and was concerned about his taking dental X-rays. He told me a story about another patient of his—she had also been trying for two years. He told her to 'take the summer off.' He was so proud of himself to have thought that up! Of course, *she* got pregnant. I got more and more uncomfortable and more and more angry; he was implying that infertility was all in my mind! I'll never go back to him again." This experience confirmed her worst fears.

These kinds of situations come up all the time as infertile couples feel the need to explain and defend themselves against the ideas that other people have. It's no wonder you want to hide away. In chapter 9, we talk about how to handle these kinds of predicaments.

The inherently sexual nature of reproductive difficulties also adds to the impulse to avoid sharing your experience. For some, talking with family members is a natural outlet, but for others, discussing sex or problems of a sexual nature is taboo. "I couldn't possibly discuss this with my parents," said Thomas, who has been trying to have a baby with his wife Leah for three years. "I know that they would be terribly upset; they want grandchildren more than anything. What I would really want from them is to give me support, to just listen. But knowing them, they would try to give me advice and fix the problem. That would make me feel more like a kid than I already do. Also, aside from the cursory, obligatory discussion about the birds and the bees when I was a teenager, we have never discussed my sexual life, and to do so now would feel weird."

Unfortunately, silence also exists—frequently and painfully—between the infertile couple. In chapter 7, we discuss the impact of infertility on your significant relationship. For now, suffice it to say that the silence often is protective in nature. Not wanting to hurt the other person or bring up painful issues, couples often avoid talking about the very things that need to be communicated most. The silence, however, can be deadly to the relationship, making matters worse.

The irony about the silence that impedes discussing infertility, whether it is with our partner, friends, family or professionals, is that in our isolation, we may become even more insecure. Our sense of being alone gives us evidence (albeit not necessarily sound) that we have failed; everyone else can do this but us. No wonder we want to hide and nurse our wounds in private.

Healing Our Self-Esteem

Just as the body needs to heal from a virus, the psyche needs to heal from a narcissistic wound. Because narcissistic wounds are not visible, they can be harder to identify, harder to know how to treat, and consequently, harder to nurse back to health. But they can heal.

A case in point is Fran, a thirty-one-year-old college administrator, who has been struggling with infertility for two years. Well-liked by students and staff, she is someone who from all outward appearances one would never suspect of feeling bad about herself. Yet even the most seemingly self-assured person is not invulnerable to narcissistic injury.

"I'm having a good day today," she announced enthusiastically. "Maybe it's because my husband suggested a vacation in Hawaii."

But with that comment, her bubble of optimism burst. Her face grew dark and sad. "I couldn't possibly go to Hawaii. I am so fat and ugly. There is no way I can get into a bathing suit—ever again."

Any good feelings she had had about herself dissolved into self-criticism—and harsh self-criticism at that. She didn't stop at feeling badly about her looks; she lamented about co-workers she was convinced didn't like her, her boss whom she felt was no longer satisfied with her work, and her friends that she was sure were avoiding her.

Fran stopped midsentence and suddenly burst into tears. "It's my husband," she exclaimed. "What if he stops loving me because I can't give him a baby?"

Fran went from feeling good to feeling lousy in the blink of an eye. What happened? How is it that Fran's strong self-esteem and positive mood evaporated so quickly? How do you hold yourself together when everything feels so wrong?

What we learn from Fran is how important it is to identify and label what has occurred. Key to the process of healing your narcissistic wounds is bringing what has been hidden in the unconscious to the forefront of your attention, to understand what the "injury" really is. So for Fran, as it is for many of our clients, it was essential to dig beneath the surface of her sudden mood swing to get to the heart of the matter. Fran's distress that day stemmed from not being able to have a baby. Infertility was at the root of her pain; infertility was the source of her self-denigration.

Because infertility attacks your core and makes you doubt your sense of self, it creeps into all facets of your life. Even though you may struggle to repress your bad feelings, it's important for you to see when and how they crop up. If you give yourself the time and space to get at the root of your anxieties, you may well find that infertility is the cause.

We also find that emotionally compartmentalizing infertility is essential to healing your sense of self. In other words, you need to put infertility in its own psychological "container," fasten the lid, and isolate it from the rest of who you are. To do this, you need to define infertility as something physical, and therefore separate from who you are as a person. Rather than thinking of infertility as if your *entire* self is flawed (both physically and emotionally), you need to view it as a *part* of your physical body that is not working correctly. If Fran had a broken arm or needed to wear glasses, would she still worry that her husband would no longer love her? Of course not, but because the effects of infertility are so pervasive, it is difficult to keep perspective so we question the very essence of who we are.

In addition to compartmentalizing the physical aspects of infertility, you need to disconnect it from your other strengths and assets. As it was for Fran, infertility makes it easy to forget that you have any skills whatsoever, but it is vitally important to bear in mind that you are more than your infertility. Remembering that you are a multifaceted and complex person, with numerous accomplishments and strengths, can help revive your healthy narcissism.

It takes work and conscious effort to remember your strong points, but doing so will allow you to feel good about yourself once again. When Fran listed her positive attributes, she gained a different perspective on her infertility trauma—she was able to separate the *worries* about herself from the *actual knowledge* of herself.

It's even helpful to write down a list of your positive attributes. Are you a good cook, athletic, creative, industrious? Are you artistic, conscientious, intelligent, funny? Are you sensitive, generous, caring, persistent? Don't be modest as you record your good qualities. Even though you may not be able to feel positive all the time, having evidence of your positive characteristics—even putting the list up on your refrigerator—is a great reminder to counteract the negative feelings that seep in. We can repair the damage to our self-esteem by giving ourselves credit where credit is due, and recognizing the strengths that we have.

So how do we heal? First, by appreciating the depth of the narcissistic damage that infertility can cause. Second, by acknowledging that your reproductive story isn't what you hoped it would be. Third, by understanding the myths and cultural pressures that make you feel less than whole, and less than others. Finally, by realizing what makes you more than your infertility. Acknowledge and celebrate your assets and strengths. Separate infertility from the rest of who you are. The more you are able to understand what happens when you suffer a narcissistic injury and the more you can compartmentalize infertility, the better and quicker you can regain your sense of self-esteem.

Just as your body recovers from a virus, your psyche can recover from the trauma of infertility. It might not be easy and it might take time—perhaps more time than you would like—but it *is* possible. You *will* feel better.

Six

Men Have Feelings Too

Men are just as vulnerable as women are to strong and difficult feelings about infertility, miscarriages, or any other reproductive trauma. Yet too often, people think that men don't have feelings about all this, or even if they do, that their feelings are basically alike and fairly simple. This assumption is incredibly off base. And as a result men are too rarely asked how they're feeling about what's going on. Everyone focuses instead on the woman's plight.

Craig calls it the "don't ask, don't tell" problem. "If you don't ask me how I feel," he said, "I certainly won't tell you. After a while, I'll start to think I'm not supposed to have feelings myself, that I'm just supposed to be supportive of my wife. Eventually, I get numb, and I forget I actually *do* have feelings—about the delays, the periods that come when you hope they won't, the tests of whether my sperm are any good, everything. But since nobody asks, even my male friends, I think there's something wrong with me for dwelling on any of this."

Men do have feelings—lots of them. They feel frustrated and angry at not being able to take control of the situation. They feel helpless and vulnerable when they can't readily fix the problem on their own, without outside help from doctors and medicine. They feel ashamed and less manly when they can't get their partner pregnant, even if no male factor is involved. When there is a male factor reason for infertility, a man's ego often takes a beating.

Men also get scared—and may be scared even to admit it. A man can feel depleted and worn-out by the ups and downs of infertility treatment, and may feel impatient when his wife needs support, especially if his own emotional needs are dismissed. Men feel the longing for a family—just as much as women do—and must grieve the loss as well.

In this chapter, we explore how men can identify their reproductive stories, and acknowledge the sadness, loss, and traumatic reactions they experience. We also discuss some uncomfortable situations for men, including:

- the infertility evaluation and dealing with the doctor— whose equipment really counts
- learning more than you wanted to know about a woman's reproductive system
- coping with shots—being an active participant in treatment
- how to be your partner's caretaker, yet not sacrifice yourself to that role

Men's Reproductive Stories

As we discussed in chapter 2, not just women have reproductive stories. Although women often respond to the idea of their story more readily than men, with a little prompting, men discover that they, too, have thoughts and feelings about having kids.

Many men *know* they will be dads someday, but they may not think too much about when or with whom. It is just a given—that's what they're supposed to do. Other men give it more conscious attention. They may know they want their first child by age thirty, they may think about having two kids, and they may hope for a daddy's girl or imagine a rough-and-tumble little boy.

Still other men may not be sure. They may want kids someday, but feel reluctant because of the enormous responsibility it entails. Sometimes men feel persuaded to have kids because their partner wants to start a family. This ambivalence can be disastrous, especially if infertility becomes an issue. Sidney, in his early forties, thought his doubts might have caused the infertility. He felt tremendous guilt that he had been undecided about starting a family.

And many men will talk about the irony of infertility after years of worrying about an accidental pregnancy. "I have spent years trying *not* to get someone pregnant," Kenneth said. "A couple of college buddies went through hell when their girlfriends got pregnant. One wound up marrying the girl, which lasted about three years. The other guy—they had an abortion; he was very supportive and it seemed they both agreed, but soon afterward they broke up. I never wanted to have to deal with it, but to be honest, in the heat of the moment . . . what I'd be thinking about had *nothing* to do with making a baby." For most men, sex is more about pleasure, a feeling of release or closeness with a partner, than it is about the possibility of reproduction.

But Kenneth, in spite of the heat of those moments, had always been cautious. He took a deep breath and added, "Now after a year and a half of no birth control, it makes me wonder if I ever had to worry in the first place."

Just as for women, men's ideas about being a parent begin in childhood. Little boys mimic their dads: they may tromp around in Daddy's shoes, talk about becoming big and strong like Dad, try to help Dad fix stuff, or pretend they are going off to work. But little boys also mimic their mothers, and this, too, becomes part of their reproductive story. Sometimes grown men forget about having cuddled or scolded their stuffed animals. Kenneth was amazed at what he remembered when he started thinking about his reproductive story. "I had three plastic dolphins that I carted with me everywhere—they were all different sizes and I made them into a mommy, a daddy, and a baby. They did circus acts in the bathtub every night, and then I tucked them into bed next to me."

Kenneth joked about getting in touch with his "feminine side," but memories like these, hidden away and out of sight for years, exist for most men. So as you start contemplating your reproductive story, think about your childhood, favorite activities, and favorite toys, as well as memories of your parents, both good and bad. More specifically, to help you reconstruct the early stages of your reproductive story, consider these questions:

- What kinds of things did you do with your father?
- What personality traits did you derive from each parent?
- Do you remember as a younger person (or now) thinking how you wanted to be similar to or different from your father or mother?
- Did you ever picture what kind of things you'd do as a father with your child, like go on hikes with the baby in a

backpack, coach Little League, repair old cars, be a Boy Scout leader, go to the fifth grade dance with your daughter, interrogate the young men she dates, and so on?

As you reflect on these questions, also consider the feelings and the nature of the connections you felt or didn't feel with your parents. What parenting has meant to you in the past influences how you think about being a parent. It's also important to think about whether you wanted to repeat the good parts or avoid the bad parts of the past when you were unconsciously scripting your reproductive story.

Men may deny having a reproductive story at first—they may not be used to thinking or talking about such things. But what we have found is that when encouraged, they open up and express their thoughts about children (beyond their fears of unwanted pregnancies), their recollections about their own childhood, and what they imagine it will be like to be a father someday.

The Dreaded Evaluation

After the requisite year of trying, feeling beaten down by not getting pregnant, a couple turns with hope, dread, excitement, and embarrassment to an infertility specialist. For both men and women, this is a turning point in their reproductive stories. "Never did I imagine I would be going to *this* kind of a doctor," said Russell, a forty-year-old businessman. It goes against the grain for men to ask for help—think about all the jokes about men asking for directions—and to seek help because something so fundamental, so easy for others, is not working right feels like a real defeat.

"I've always prided myself on my physical strength," Russell continued. "Even when I was exhausted, I've worked long hours—just to get the job done. It's what's got me where I am today. Yet working hard hasn't helped much with having a baby. I just can't get my wife pregnant."

Russell's comment stands out in sharp contrast to others who say, "*We* can't get pregnant." It is, after all, a joint effort. His sense of sole responsibility, even before a diagnosis has been determined, is not uncommon. Many men connect infertility with commonplace male doubts about adequacy and functioning in the sexual arena, especially related to the size or functioning of their genitals. It is rare that a woman will complain, "He can't get me pregnant," even when the infertility is due to a male factor. Most often, the blame and guilt comes from a man's internal sense of shame, not from his partner.

Men often focus on their individual achievements; they pride themselves on their accomplishments. When the male *is* the one responsible for the couple's infertility, and thus interprets this as his inability to "get the job done," it's not surprising that feelings of shame and inadequacy are so overwhelming. Just as it is important for a woman to separate her sense of self from her ability to get pregnant, a man needs to remind himself that getting a woman pregnant does not define his identity, his manliness, or, ultimately, his "fatherliness."

When an infertile man starts to think negatively and compares himself to other men who easily have children, we like to remind him that George Washington, the "father" of our country, memorialized by a huge, phallic obelisk in the city named after him, was unable to have children with his wife. Although we don't know for certain, George probably had male factor infertility because

Martha had four children by her previous marriage. Yet nobody thinks of him as less masculine or less heroic because of this.

The Doctor's Equipment Works, but Mine Doesn't

Turning to a fertility specialist is rife with feelings for both men and women. The intrusion of third parties into a couple's intimate life can be embarrassing and uncomfortable. Seeking help means you are admitting to yourself and to a stranger that you are in need. This is rarely easy to divulge, and may be more difficult for a man than for a woman, since men tend to want to solve problems on their own, rather than admitting their need for help.

A man may feel a particular threat if he makes a comparison between himself and the potency of the infertility specialist's medical magic. Anthony, a thirty-five-year-old scientist at an infertility evaluation, was reluctant to reveal his difficulties. He said, "This doctor and a bunch of technicians will get her pregnant, when I can't." He felt diminished in his capacity as a man and a bit competitive with the doctor. So during the evaluation, he felt compelled to impress the doctor with his knowledge of technology. The doctor, delighted to have someone to talk shop with, tried to engage Anthony by discussing the laboratory equipment and other high-tech gadgets in his office. Though the doctor meant well, Anthony felt a resurgence of shame. "All this equipment belongs to *him,* not me, and we only need it because *my* 'equipment' isn't working!"

Sometimes, the chemistry between a doctor and patient really isn't right—for men as well as women—whether a consultation is for infertility or any other medical problem. If you find this to be the case, it's okay to follow your gut reaction and get a second opinion—in fact, it may be crucial to do so in order to make the whole process tolerable. If, however, you find that these feelings of inadequacy exist with all the infertility specialists you consult, it may have more to do with you than with the doctor.

Sometimes the feelings of competition and shame in relation to the doctor can be reduced if men can think of their physician as a colleague or teammate. No one would dream of climbing Mt. Everest without a support group, without food, oxygen, or the right tools. And as anybody who's been there knows, infertility can feel like the steepest mountain in the world. Your doctor is on the climb too, and will work with you, not against you.

To achieve your objective of having a family, remind yourself that doctors are not the enemy. They are not there to pass judgment or criticize, nor do they intend to dominate or diminish your manliness. Think of it this way: you are merely borrowing their knowledge, their "equipment," and their support to reach your final goal.

Nerve-wracking Tests

Unless a man needs to go through a surgical procedure to obtain his sperm, the bulk of the testing falls on the woman. She will have multiple procedures, like having blood levels drawn, endometrial biopsies, any number of surgeries, painful daily shots, and reactions to hormonal medications. Still, although a woman may be subjected to more procedures, all of them are expressly medical. While less invasive than most of the procedures that women face, the uniquely male procedure—having to produce a semen specimen for analysis—is more directly sexual. Masturbating on demand is hardly the same as masturbating for pleasure, but it is sexual nonetheless.

It can also be absurd and embarrassing. At his first urology appointment, the nurse sent Murray to the bathroom to produce a semen sample. "Not only did it take a while to get things going," he said, "but I missed the specimen cup! I'm standing there with my pants around my ankles, specimen cup in one hand, you know what in the other. What the hell was I supposed to do then? And if things weren't bad enough, I had to explain it all to the nurse."

Although Murray laughed about it later, underneath his storytelling were painful feelings of shame. Though the nurse had been very professional, Murray was reminded of mistakes he had made, including his mother's anger and his brother's taunts for missing the toilet when he was a little boy. As his semen was analyzed, Murray felt his old self-doubts reactivated. In his mind, the count, morphology, and motility of his sperm translated into "there aren't enough, they are deformed, and they can't swim to save their lives."

Men can cope with the anxiety and strain of these experiences in several ways. First, finding humor in this absurd situation helps to relieve some tension. More importantly, it helps to realize you're not alone. There's relief in acknowledging, sharing, and receiving validation for feelings of shame and humiliation. Hearing what other men in similar situations have experienced can be helpful on many levels. Every man who has gone through infertility testing has his own version of the bathroom story to tell.

"It helped me to talk to other guys," Murray said, "because I realized that they weren't aliens or geeks or weird in any way. They were just like me." Talking about it can help remind you that your feelings are normal, and that everyone feels humiliated and embarrassed by these tests.

Infertility and Your Relationship

Acknowledging that infertility affects your relationship with your partner may qualify as the understatement of the century! The real question is what part of your relationship *doesn't* it affect? The anxiety, the financial strain, the physical demands, the blow to egos, and lest we forget, the tensions it creates in the bedroom—all this takes its toll on a couple. In this section, we explore the different ways men may respond to the strain infertility imposes, and offer suggestions of how to cope.

A Woman's Anatomy—More than You Ever Thought You'd Know

Infertility forces men to pay more attention to the female reproductive system than ever before. Women, who have had to deal with their menstrual cycle since early adolescence, are used to the physical shifts that occur monthly—the cramps, the bloating, the blood. But men aren't. Even sensitive and mature men can be surprisingly squeamish and ignorant about menstruation. They may think of menstruation in terms of moodiness and sensitivity, irritability, messiness, and as an interruption in sexual activity. When infertility hits, however, a man is forced to confront and deal with a woman's body in ways that weren't necessary before.

Some men cope by making a scientific project out of monitoring temperature to know the exact timing of ovulation, assessing changes in vaginal mucus, and charting the starting day of each menstrual cycle. While this helps some men by giving them an active role in the process, others feel odd about taking an interest in all of the "female stuff" they previously avoided. This often depends on how much exposure you may have had growing up.

"Being the only son and growing up with three older sisters," Jerry said, "there were always boxes of tampons and pads in the bathroom. Someone was always talking about how awful they were feeling at that time of the month." Because of his early family experiences, Jerry was quite at ease talking about these issues with his wife and their doctor.

Clark wasn't. "I feel bad admitting this," he said, "but the whole thing grosses me out." As a teenager, Clark had to empty the wastebaskets. "It was disgusting. I remember bloody sanitary napkins in the garbage. I don't know why my mother didn't wrap them up." Whenever Clark's wife wanted to talk to him about her cycle, he would involuntarily cringe. "I know we're in this infertility treatment together," he said, "but I don't want to know all the nitty-gritty details."

Wherever you are on the continuum, from comfort with female biology to avoidance of it, talking about it with your partner can help your relationship. If she understands why certain things bother or embarrass you, she can be more sensitive to your needs. Clark's wife, once she realized how easily upset he was by menstrual blood and feminine hygiene products, minimized his exposure to them. She also understood why he avoided them and no longer took it personally; thus, he was more supportive because he knew she understood.

The Shots
This treatment phase is agonizing for both men and women— and not for the same reasons. For women, the shots hurt. "I hate

needles," Trish moaned. "I almost passed out when I realized I was going to have daily injections—and into my abdomen, of all places!" For men who are giving their partners shots, a range of emotions may emerge: from feeling positive in his newfound role as an active participant to feelings of dread as the one inflicting pain.

Artie fell into the positive category. "I felt so bad for my wife— she was the one being subjected to so much. All I had to do was give the semen sample, but she's had one test after another. So, in a weird way, I feel good that I can help with the shots. At least I'm doing something." After feeling peripheral to the treatment process, Artie felt re-engaged with his wife and joked about playing doctor with her. Giving the shots took away some of the helplessness he had been feeling, gave him a renewed feeling of competence, and allowed him to do something active regarding treatment. After months or years of mounting tension about infertility, giving the shots allows some men to reconnect with their wives as teammates, and couples to experience this treatment phase together.

Other men respond quite differently. Colin tried to seem stoic when he received instructions on how to administer the shots. "The nurse showed me how to do it when we were at the doctor's office, then sent me home with a printout of the steps I had to follow. It looked straightforward enough, but when it was time for us to do it at home, I was shaking like a leaf. The instructions said to insert the needle quickly, like a dart. I was standing there, pinching Adie's skin, needle ready to go, and I couldn't do it. I froze. Meanwhile, Adie was lying on the bed, getting more and more impatient. She said, 'Just do it already!' And so I did, and she started to cry, and then I got angry. I knew I hurt her and I felt terrible about it, but I was doing the best that I could and I didn't think she appreciated that. I shouted, 'Maybe you should get somebody else to do this!' and that's when we really started arguing."

Colin quickly realized that they were depleted—from the shots but also from all the months of procedures and disappointments. It wasn't only the physical act of giving the shots, but what the shots represented. He felt so guilty after their argument; he brought flowers home. He joked that their condo would soon look like a florist if he had to bring home flowers every time he gave Adie her shots.

It's all too easy to forget that it's emotionally stressful to give the shots, as well as to receive them. It can sometimes help to give the first shot in the doctor's office, with a nurse's support and guidance. Any tricks you can use to make giving shots easier are fine. Josh worried about getting the progesterone shots in the right spot, especially after one particularly painful injection came too close to a nerve. He and his wife felt much more comfortable after he drew a circle in permanent marker on his wife's hip so he knew exactly where to aim.

For Colin, it helped to know he wasn't alone in his apprehension. Some men can't administer the shots because of their anxiety, and their partner must either find another person to help or learn to give herself the shots. In other cases, women don't want their partners to give them the shots, preferring to maintain control of the situation themselves. This can leave the man feeling like an unnecessary appendage. It can make men feel even more emasculated—as if "here's one more thing you can't get right."

What's most important as you struggle with this phase of treatment is to keep perspective on what is really going on. The shots and the tensions they arouse reflect the strain that infertility imposes on a relationship. Reminding yourself of this each time you pick up that syringe can help you keep your focus on the big picture.

Male Factor Treatment: No Picnic Either

Although women typically bear the brunt of the invasive diagnostic and treatment methods when going through infertility, men are not far behind. Male factor problems account for 40 percent of infertility, and recently the treatment of male factors has burgeoned. Male factor infertility can be due to low sperm count, poor sperm motility, poor sperm quality, or sperm that are not able to penetrate the egg. Autoimmune reactions, female allergies to male semen, and vasectomies that cannot be successfully reversed are also problems couples encounter.

Medical procedures now available offer hope to couples with male factor infertility. ICSI (intracytoplasmic sperm injection), TESA (testicular sperm aspiration), and TESE (testicular sperm extraction) are a few of the advances in interventions for men. While ICSI sperm can be obtained through masturbation, some of the other methods require that sperm be obtained surgically, either under conscious sedation or general anesthetic.

While very promising, these procedures can be extremely anxiety-provoking. The tendency for a man to associate his sense of self, masculinity, and competence with his genitals makes him especially vulnerable to psychological injury from these procedures. Normal, early childhood fears of castration can be re-evoked when a man faces genital surgery. Little boys protect themselves from their fears by arming themselves with superhero capes and pirate swords. Grown men may worry that their "equipment" is damaged, confirming their childhood fantasies, or that it could be hurt by a procedure.

These fears add to men's sense of vulnerability, making them feel even less manly. These fears and feelings are normal. It is helpful for a man to compartmentalize his medical needs from the rest of him, and actively use his cognitive and analytical skills to separate the medical procedure from his personal identity.

Sex as Baby-making, Not Lovemaking

Men also need to be reassured that in most cases their partner is not looking at them as a baby-making machine. When women are asked if they've considered trading in their partner because of infertility, most look shocked and say, "Of course not!"

Cara, whose husband had a low sperm count and low motility, said, "I married the guy because I love him, and I still do—no matter what. Being able to make a baby has nothing to do with what kind of father I know Jamie will be. We're just going to have to take a different path to becoming parents."

While most men don't complain if their partner shows an increased interest in sex, things can get more complicated when the upsurge is due to wanting a baby. You may feel that she is more interested in someone or something other than you, and that sex has gone from being a sensuous act of love to a practical "manufacturing" task. It may feel as if you are being used, almost as if you are only good for one thing.

Graham, a thirty-five-year-old general contractor, described feeling left out of lovemaking when he and his wife had sex. "I think part of it is because we are on a schedule," he said. "It's not like it used to be. It's not like, 'Hey, hon, are you in the mood?' It's more like, 'It's Tuesday, gotta do it.' I know it's not easy for my wife either, but I have to admit, I feel like I'm a faucet that gets used for doing the dishes."

Graham feels dehumanized by the timetable of sex. One of the worst negative side effects of infertility treatment is this impact on the couple's sex life. It's good to keep in mind that this phase of your relationship, the baby-making years, will not go on forever.

Some Things Can't be Fixed

For many men, the most debilitating aspect of infertility is that they can't *do* anything to make it better. Men like to take action; they repair things, take control, and try to make things right. This is not to say that men aren't reflective and thoughtful, it's just that when there's a problem, their natural response is to fix it. The conundrum is that infertility is a problem that you can't just fix—not easily—and usually not without medical assistance. You may feel helpless, not only because you can't make a baby, but also because you can't help your partner stop feeling sad.

"Every time Heidi cries," Jonathan said, "my stomach ties up in knots. I never know what to do. I know I'm supposed to be a sensitive and liberated modern male who understands the value of just listening. But there are times when I'm fed up with it all. I'm tired of listening to her talk about who else got pregnant or what she's read on the Internet. But mostly I'm tired of her tears because there's nothing I can do to stop them." Jonathan felt inadequate not only because, as he added, "Every other guy has kids and I don't," but also because he didn't know how to handle Heidi's intense waves of emotion.

Men as Caretakers

Men can take the helpless feelings that Jonathan described and translate them into taking care of their partners. As we discussed earlier, some men feel empowered by administering the shots. Other men make sure that they attend every doctor's appointment or they take control of the financial and insurance aspects of treatment. Being actively involved in making sure *she's* okay, allows *him* to feel better too.

As long as your wife does not feel belittled and forced into a needy or helpless role, she can certainly benefit from your support. If it helps you to feel more in control—especially since so much control slips away with infertility—putting energy into caretaking can be a way for you to regain some sense of effectiveness and restore some aspects of your masculine identity. Some men, however, become overly focused on the pragmatic side of infertility treatment as a way of avoiding their emotions. They hide their vulnerable side—which they don't want to expose—behind a driven determination to take action and avoid passivity at all costs. Many men tend to avoid sad feelings and grief because it feels weak to have such feelings. Sitting and "just talking" can be similarly anxiety provoking.

"Marie is always nagging me to talk," complained Rob. "Why can't she realize that it makes me feel terrible to just sit there and not be able to do anything?"

"But you keep me at such a distance," Marie responded. "You never let me in or let me help. It makes me feel like you don't value or trust what I could offer."

The problem with driven activity and excessive caretaking is that they keep your own feelings from ever being resolved because you deny them, even to yourself. Further, it robs your wife of the chance to gain strength by being helpful to you for a change, and of the chance to feel connected with you by understanding what you feel.

Women don't always grasp this need that men have to feel in control of their own emotions and situations. Your wife may feel, as you throw yourself into aspects of the treatment in a matter-of-fact fashion, that you don't care or have any feelings about this trauma, because you are not expressing them in a way she understands. Because you are not letting your feelings out the way she does, she may get angry and be unappreciative of your caretaking efforts. You may think, *What more does she want? I'm doing everything I can!*

As we discuss in chapter 7, men and women cope very differently, especially when under stress. If you can educate your partner as to how you cope best, she will realize that you really do have feelings, and that you are trying to cope as best as you can, just as she is.

Feeling Angry

The traumas and losses of infertility treatment, like most other traumas and losses, lead not only to feelings of sadness and grief, but also to intense anger that people—and especially men—don't know what to do with. Duncan and Beatrice have been trying for six years, with multiple failed IVFs. Beatrice's depression over infertility has depleted her energy and drive. "I try to shut out all the infertility stuff when I'm at work, but as soon as I get home, I can feel that dark gloom over everything," Duncan said. "She's either silent, or crying, or she barks at me. I get tired of it sometimes. And forget it, if I have something else to talk about, if an issue came up at work for me. That makes me want to bark back. Then I feel like a jerk."

Some of the anger men feel is the natural result of the traumatic and stressful circumstances surrounding infertility. For many men, however, their situational anger is compounded by the revival of feelings from earlier times in their lives. Duncan experienced both. The oldest of three, he resented the attention his mother always seemed to be paying to his younger siblings. So Beatrice's intense focus on having a baby made him feel secondary, once again, to the most important woman in his life. Understanding that Beatrice's attention to infertility had nothing to do with her feelings toward him helped Duncan to keep his past and present separate. After Beatrice reassured him of his significance as her partner and the future father of their kids, his anger dissipated.

Men can deal with their anger and frustration in other ways as well. Sometimes they need to blow off steam. One weekend, after a particularly stressful afternoon of listening to his wife rant about her sister's just-announced pregnancy, Richard was beside himself. "I listened, I consoled, I did as much as I could, but as the day wore on, I wore out. I didn't unleash on Akiko, although there were moments when I had to bite my tongue, but after she calmed down, I went to the batting cages with my brother," Richard said. "After smashing a few dozen balls and then talking with Jim, I felt exhausted, but calmer." Releasing his own anger through physical activity gave Richard renewed energy to support his wife during this particular crisis.

Hidden Grief

Of course, men do not only feel anger and resentment. As we have seen, they feel anxious and scared, out of control, embarrassed by their ineffectiveness (even if the infertility is *not* caused by male factor), and terribly sad. Their sadness is due to the many losses and the unexpected changes in their reproductive stories, the loss of their views of themselves as masculine and strong, the loss of intimacy that infertility so insidiously steals, as well as the loss of the sense that they are like all the other men out there who are dads.

The problem that comes up for couples, then, is not that men don't have feelings, but that they often do not reveal them in the ways that women do. Women are more likely to show depression and grief in easily recognizable ways: they cry and readily confess they are sad and in pain. They are generally more open about saying they are depressed, and more likely to seek help—by talking to friends, joining a support group, reading books, or going to therapy.

Since men don't necessarily open up the same way, people—even their wives—often don't realize that they too are suffering. For many men, the most unmanly thing of all is to admit the feelings of sadness, grief and helplessness that accompany infertility.

So how do men grieve and deal with the other feelings that go along with infertility? For many men, profound sadness and tears only come out rarely, and usually when they are alone. More typically, they reveal their feelings in less direct ways. As we have seen, many men attempt to handle feelings by going into "action mode" in some area of their lives unrelated to infertility. Sometimes they throw themselves into work. If they can't feel accomplished in the reproductive part of their lives, they can at least glean success at something they do have control over, namely work. Other men exercise more when they are upset. At least they can make their bodies function properly in *this* way. These can be constructive and adaptive ways of dealing with stress and grief unless it becomes obsessive or takes you away from other important aspects of your life, including your relationship with your wife.

Still other men build things. Ted and his wife, Sharon, had a miscarriage at fourteen weeks after getting pregnant with IVF, and this was after four years of various interventions. Returning from the hospital after Sharon had a D&C, Ted tore out all the kitchen cabinets, ripped up the old linoleum, and removed the kitchen sink. "It all needed to get done sometime," he said. Sharon, recuperating from the surgery and loss, was stunned and wanted to know why now?

Ted, not conscious of his motives at the time, later came to realize that this was part of his grief. "I was so angry, the demolition work let me take it out physically. My baby died and I had to do something." Ted also had a need to feel he could create something new. He didn't have control over the miscarriage or all those years of infertility, so he put his energy into something he did have control over. He could rebuild the kitchen even if he couldn't have a baby.

Unfortunately, sometimes men handle their feelings by throwing themselves into alcohol, drugs, or other self-destructive behavior. Drowning one's sorrow and pain in drink or other forms of self-medication is, obviously, not in your best interests. It may temporarily blunt your feelings, but never does it help you get over them. In fact, it usually causes more harm and adds another level of trauma the couple must contend with.

Seven

Relationships Under Fire

I remember exactly when I fell in love with Stephanie. She had invited me over for dinner. I was watching her puttering around the kitchen and I suddenly had this picture of us as married and that we had just put our kids to bed. I was so happy. It was such a simple moment but one that changed my life. I don't understand what is happening to us now. It's so different from what I pictured. —Eric, after two years of infertility

Infertility is not just an individual trauma. The stress that the experience places on your relationship can leave you feeling that you're alone in this, not facing this crisis together as partners, as a team. The very person you want to feel closest to may seem to be pulling away. Not only do you each have to deal with the trauma individually, you also must cope with how your partner is coping. And, like Eric, you must also come to terms with how your shared reproductive story is changing.

We've said this before but it bears repeating: infertility takes its toll on all intimate relationships. So the problems you may be experiencing as a couple most likely don't stem from your relationship but from the enormous stress caused by infertility. Couples must remember—and be reminded—that they each go through this reproductive trauma in their own way. Yet, if you do not understand how each of you copes, you may take your differences in coping and reactions personally, feeling that "if my partner really loved me, she or he wouldn't act this way."

Even though both of you may feel helpless, guilty, inadequate—all the difficult feelings we've been discussing—you are not clones of each other, and you handle these feelings in different ways. Infertility may be the toughest test your relationship has had to endure so far—and you have to learn and work on the skills that can help you come closer, not drift further apart.

What Is Happening to Us?

"I was four days late this month," said Roseanne. "My breasts were very swollen and sore and I felt exhausted. I really thought this might be it." Roseanne and her husband, Glenn, were in the midst of an infertility workup and still trying on their own. When her period started, Roseanne turned to Glenn for support. He, understanding of how sad she was—once again—let her cry, gave her a big hug, then started talking about the lunch meeting he had with his boss that day. That's when she lost it. "He just switched gears on me," she cried. "Sometimes I think he doesn't care!"

Glenn does care; he just doesn't feel his grief the same way Roseanne does. For Roseanne, the experience is physical—she feels the hormonal shifts and mood changes, feels the changes in her body, feels the cramps of a menstrual cycle. She has to deal with blood and tampons and pads, which under normal circumstances is an annoyance, but with infertility marks a significant loss. Glenn's experience is much less immediate; he is physically removed from it, and as we discussed in chapter 6, some men shy away from the biological aspects of the female reproductive system anyway.

When you experience infertility you may worry terribly when you find yourself in conflict with your partner, at a time when you need each other desperately. Roseanne didn't understand what she interpreted as Glenn's indifference. She wanted to talk and be reassured, which Glenn attempted, but from her perspective it wasn't enough. Yet for Glenn to cope, he needed to move on, because dwelling on the feelings—or the topic—made him feel worse. What he wanted more than anything was to fix the infertility, but this he couldn't repair. So he switched the topic. And both Roseanne and Glenn, each still hurting inside, hurt each other with their different coping styles.

We see this with couples time and again: a disconnect between the couple since their coping styles are at odds. It can happen with each failed monthly cycle. It can happen over financial matters that affect treatment decisions. It can also happen when any decision about treatment needs to be made, such as how many IVF cycles to try, whether to use donor eggs or sperm, or whether or not to adopt.

Differences of opinion are to be expected, but what's crucial during this extremely stressful time is how you negotiate through divergent feelings with your partner. Because you and your partner may cope with stress differently, understanding how your partner responds, and vice versa, gives you the opportunity to navigate these rough waters together, rather than feeling alone and adrift at sea.

How Do *You* Cope?

When you are overwhelmed emotionally, what do you do? Are you a talker or do you process your feelings privately? Do you lash out or internalize anger? Do you work more when you're stressed or less? Does exercise help, or would you rather relax in front of the TV? What happens when you feel out of control? Do you become more controlling or do you relinquish control? Do you become more active or do you retreat into passivity? These are questions you and your partner can ask yourselves and each other to help you identify your personal coping styles.

Nancy, 38, and Jake, 36, recently found out that Jake has a variocele, requiring surgery. "Jake and I have always gotten along, but since he was diagnosed, he is very irritable and moody. He criticizes everything I do. I've never seen him like this." Since the diagnosis, Nancy has been researching online about this condition and sharing her findings with Jake.

"She's driving me crazy," said Jake. "It's enough already. I wish she would leave me alone. When I want to talk about it I will, but I don't want to talk about it all the time."

Are Jake's true colors coming out? Probably not. He and Nancy are both in shock, reeling from the unexpected news about his condition. Jake, understandably, feels inadequate and defective. To cope, he's retreating into himself; he wants to ponder his diagnosis and upcoming surgery privately, so Nancy's prodding feels intrusive. She, on the other hand, finds that doing research makes her feel better.

By being honest with each other about their coping styles, Jake and Nancy realized that they were dealing with the diagnosis in their own ways—and that neither method was inherently better than the other. To negotiate their way through this stressful time, they decided to be more patient with each other as well as pay more attention to what each other was saying—not just the verbal conversations, but the nonverbal cues as well. So, if Jake rolled his eyes when Nancy discovered a new article to read, instead of taking it personally, she would put it on his night table to look at when he wanted. Similarly, Jake made a point of thanking Nancy for finding the article and telling her what he thought after he read it.

Nancy and Jake are typical of many couples—where one person benefits from talking about the next step, while the other needs to process it internally. Like Nancy, you may need to research every option in great detail, while your partner may feel overwhelmed by the information.

It's also startling when you've been on the same page regarding treatment decisions, but as time goes on and spirits deflate, tensions build over difficult decisions and you suddenly find yourselves at an impasse. When Eric reminisced about falling in love with Stephanie, and pictured tucking his kids in at night, he was dismayed at how far afield his dreams had come. Up until this point in their nine years of marriage, Stephanie and Eric were able to compromise and negotiate when stressful situations occurred. Running a real estate business together had given them plenty of practice in this. Yet now, after two years of using Clomid and attempting four IUIs, they argue constantly about what to do next. Stephanie wants to try an IVF cycle, but Eric isn't sure it's worth it. "I want kids, but the statistics for IVF are not encouraging," Eric said. "It doesn't seem like the best investment."

Stephanie bristled when she heard this. "I can't believe all he can think about is money. How can he be so rigid and closed minded at a time like this?"

At their low points, Stephanie wonders if Eric is the right man after all, and Eric is confused by feeling so disconnected from his wife. Just as an individual can suffer a narcissistic injury, so can a couple. Stephanie and Eric's conflict over trying IVF and spending so much money made them doubt what they had always believed: that they were soul mates, that they would make good parents, that they were a team.

What feels like an impossible impasse in their relationship doesn't have to do with their closeness as a couple; the circumstances of their infertility have thrown them off course. Their individual ways of dealing with stress—he the logical thinker, she more emotionally driven—have always been part of their attraction to each other, to say nothing of being an asset to their business. But now at this crossroads, their coping styles are clashing, and they are pushing each other away in hurt and anger.

When you find yourself in a similar situation, take the first step of recognizing your own coping mechanism (by asking yourself questions like those at the beginning of this section), then your partner's. Second, you must accept that both of your approaches are reasonable. If Stephanie can understand that Eric becomes analytical because he is frightened of losing control (more on this later), she will become less personally hurt. Similarly, if Eric can appreciate Stephanie's fears of not having a family, he can provide support and comfort rather than feel defensive. Likewise, you and you partner will have more empathy for each other and be better able to accept each other's differences.

Who's in Control Here Anyway?

Loss of control is one of the most uncomfortable feelings evoked by infertility. It leaves you feeling trapped, inadequate, and desperate. Imagine then if two people living together both feel that at the same time. It's pretty intense. In some cases people may try to regain a sense of control by becoming more controlling in their relationship. But while taking control in some areas of life can be a great antidote to helplessness, a way to protect yourself against feeling vulnerable, it can also interfere with your relationship with your partner.

Sometimes the need for control is an attempt to get your needs met by your partner, even at the sacrifice of his or her own needs. That's when the power struggles emerge—when you and your partner both desperately want your own needs met at the same time. During infertility, couples who previously saw themselves as teammates begin to view each other as obstacles, when that person may simply be trying to keep from drowning in his/her own feelings.

Taking control becomes a problem when you are not aware of why you are doing it. Consider Ed and Joan, both forty-two and trying to get pregnant for three years. Joan underwent two surgeries to clear her blocked fallopian tubes; they also had one failed IVF procedure. Their doctor suggested using an egg donor to improve their chances, but Joan would rather adopt. "If the baby can't be both of ours, then it should be neither of ours," she said.

While Ed expressed his willingness to proceed with adoption, it has been a struggle every step of the way. "He says he'll fill out the paperwork, and then he procrastinates," complained Joan. "If I remind him, he calls me a nag. I can't win."

"I'll do it," responded Ed. "But I'm really busy. I'll get to it when I can."

"But you're always busy with something," exclaimed Joan. "I'm beginning to think you don't even want kids!"

"You know I do. You just always need to have everything on your terms," Ed countered.

Ed finally finished the paperwork, only to find fault with the potential birth mothers who expressed interest in choosing them. Joan felt desperate to move on. When she confronted Ed, he finally admitted that his heart was not really in adoption; he wanted to try using donor eggs. "She was so adamant about adoption that I was afraid that she would leave if I didn't go along with it," he said.

Instead of being open with his feelings, Ed fell back on passive resistance—the procrastination, the vetoing—to solve his dilemma. As a result, Joan was furious and hurt. Their power struggle revolved around their needs and their fears—her need for a baby, and his fear of expressing his true feelings.

When Ed opened up to Joan, their struggle was defused. She could empathize with his anxiety, rather than combating his negative behavior. As they talked about the deeper feelings motivating them, both Ed and Joan relaxed, able to respect each other's feelings without feeling so threatened by them. As the conflict abated, Ed and Joan felt more open to the different options available to them, and agreed to use an egg donor.

Sometimes couples don't struggle for control over the big infertility issues but instead wrangle over the smaller stuff. "We really try to stay connected," said Samantha, "but sometimes Tony and I fight over the stupidest things! Where to go for dinner, or which dining room chairs we want. Everything always has to be his way or he's miserable."

"I want to feel like I have control in some tiny aspect of my life," Tony responded. "Everywhere I look, someone is telling me what to do—at work, and at home, the doctors, and everybody! Sometimes I want to be the one to decide."

Tony is understandably angry at his loss of control. The problem arises from his need to regain his sense of control at Samantha's expense. She too feels powerless about her inability to conceive, so she fights Tony to regain some sense of empowerment.

If you find yourself engaged in this kind of bickering with your partner, it helps to pause and think: *Will this decision matter in an hour? A day? A week? A month?* Most of these disagreements have no meaning in and of themselves—it doesn't really matter where you go to dinner—but they take on meaning in the moment because both of you are trying to grab hold of something to keep your heads above water in the stormy seas of your medical crisis.

Control over Money

Under the best of circumstances, money can trigger marital disputes. Couples handle money in varied ways; some pool their resources, while others keep separate bank accounts, with a shared account for household expenses. If tiffs occur over small purchases, spending large sums of money on infertility treatment will likely cause huge fights.

It can feel frightening to invest your money in infertility treatment when there are no guarantees. This anxiety may be the impetus for control battles. With Eric and Stephanie, part of his resistance to IVF stemmed from his fears of spending money. He became controlling of the situation in an attempt to manage this anxiety.

Setting a limit on how much you spend on ART works for many couples. Eric and Stephanie agreed they would try a maximum of three IVF cycles. We have found it helpful for our clients to negotiate and agree upon some of this ahead of time, even before consulting an infertility specialist if possible, so the plan is clear to both. This road map needs to be flexible, though; your feelings may change as your situation changes. We recommend that couples revisit and revise their joint agreements about finances and other treatment decisions periodically—say every few months. We explore these strategies in chapter 10, but, at this point, couples need to be aware that the financial tensions may be a conduit for all sorts of feelings about yourselves and all that you are going through.

Control in the Bedroom

During infertility, sex and reproduction become integrally entwined, as sex becomes less about pleasure and connection and more about making a baby. Sex becomes goal-directed, and that goal is ever elusive. When infertility takes center stage, medical timetables and routines can dampen the very spark needed to create a baby. This invasion of sexual intimacy can create a domino effect of loneliness and isolation by damaging each partner's self-esteem and their connection to one another.

Control issues can also crop up in the bedroom. If one partner is silently—or actively—angry with the other, or is depressed, the

gulf between them widens. Interest in sex may decline, or a partner may withhold sex to express anger. "I feel so fat and ugly, I just
don't feel sexual anymore," said Janine. "When I'm depressed, I
don't care about sex."

Janine was resistant not only because of her body image; having
sex underscored feelings of failure. Understanding this helped Janine and her partner, Oscar, reconnect. "I didn't realize that each
time I wanted sex," Oscar said, "Janine was reminded of not having a baby. I didn't connect the two—to me sex was for fun, a release, it feels good. But for her, sex isn't what it used to be." So
Janine and Oscar separated out baby-making time from lovemaking the rest of the month, a compromise that respected both of
their needs.

I Don't Want it to be My Fault

Blaming yourself, as Janine did even though the cause of their infertility couldn't be specified by her doctors, infiltrates your relationship both inside the bedroom and outside of it. If you are the
one diagnosed with the problem, you may feel guilty that you are
denying your partner the family he or she desires. In spite of all the
reassurances your partner may give you, you may still feel awful.

"I worry that Pete is going to hate me because it's all my fault,"
Megan said. Although she is only thirty-three, Megan's hormonal
levels indicate early onset of perimenopause. Pete has been supportive and caring throughout, but Megan can't shake her anxiety.
"I wonder if he thinks about being with someone else; someone
younger who wouldn't have these problems."

So Megan seeks repeated reassurances from Pete that she is the
girl of his dreams. Now that he understands her feelings, Pete has

been able to give her steady support, which has helped her separate her other good qualities from infertility. Realizing that she had little control over her body, she focused instead on what she could control.

Since guilt is a heavy feeling to carry, many people fight it off by becoming defensive or critical. Madison and Trevor, 38 and 40, were at each other about everything, from taking out the trash to taking care of finances, from exercising (she didn't think he did enough; he thought she was doing too much) to which friends they would see on the weekend. This bickering masked bitter feelings they both had about their postponing starting a family, resulting in age-related infertility and poor egg quality. Madison accused Trevor of forcing them to wait while he finished graduate school. Trevor blamed her. "Madison keeps saying I wasn't ready, but it's not true. Plus I got my degree six years ago. She didn't want to start a family until we bought a big house in the 'right' neighborhood."

When a couple finds themselves in a raging battle, it can be helpful to remember what brought you together in the first place. Stepping back from the fray, calling a truce, and reminding yourself of the qualities you love in your partner can help to lower the levels of anger and re-establish your bond. Just as individuals can suffer narcissistic injuries due to infertility, so can couples. Your sense of accomplishment as a couple mirrors your own individual sense of yourself as a healthy, whole, competent adult. When treatment continues to be unsuccessful over a long period of time, it becomes difficult to resist the relentless wearing away of your sense of self as a couple.

Madison and Trevor each had to come to grips with their previous ambivalence about having children. It is quite common and normal for people to question whether they want a family or not. But to blame each other for earlier indecision is not fair, and can be quite destructive as you push yourselves further and further apart.

When one partner is certain about wanting a baby no matter what, and the other is less sure, the couple can become engaged in a battle of wills that is not only exhausting, but almost impossible to resolve comfortably. When a couple stakes out opposite positions, decisions about infertility treatments become a battleground where one person must give in to the other. Unfortunately, a decision made under these circumstances is invariably accompanied by resentment, guilt, and anxiety. If you have acquiesced, you may be furious at being forced to relent. If you "won," you may feel indebted to your partner for relenting. None of this adds up to a healthy relationship.

Madison and Trevor resolved their differences when they realized how similar their reactions had been. They each owned up to the role they played in the delay and no longer blamed each other. "When we stopped fighting," Madison said, "we could see that *finally* we were both on the same page about having a family. It is something we both really want." Madison and Trevor eventually adopted a little boy from Korea.

Traumas and Secrets from the Past

As discussed in chapter 5, memories of past reproductive traumas can resurface during infertility. A member of a couple may feel renewed guilt and worry that their partner will judge them as they may be judging themselves. If these issues remain buried, they can fester and cause friction within the current relationship.

Theresa had dated Brian for several years before they married, and during that time they had broken up and reconciled several times. During one breakup, Theresa discovered she was pregnant with Brian's baby, and without telling Brian, she had an abortion. "At the time I thought the relationship was really over," she said. "I didn't want a baby under those circumstances, and I didn't want to involve him in the decision. When we got back together, I never could find the right time or the right words to tell him." She kept her secret because she was terrified he would leave her if he knew. Now, faced with infertility, her secret was eating at her.

Theresa decided to take a chance and tell Brian. She needed to know if he would stay with her even if she couldn't have a baby and accept her past choice. Although he was angry at first, and had to face his own grief about this past loss, he could appreciate her decision and agony over telling him. Ultimately it brought the two of them much closer together in their dealings with the current infertility.

Any unresolved grief, if it is not dealt with, accompanies you as you progress through your life. Likewise, secrets that you bear alone may be heavy burdens. Once you talk about these issues—whether with your partner or with a therapist—and work them through, it clears the way to proceed with your current challenges less encumbered.

How Can We Possibly Get Through This?

How do you get through this as a couple? First, know that you can. Yes, the stresses of infertility challenge the most solid bonds and your relationship is undergoing a severe test as are both of you individually. But recognizing and acknowledging this gives you room to gain greater insight into how your infertility trauma is affecting both you and your partner. Second, we counsel couples to focus on two key tools: communication—being open with each other—and negotiation—so you can accommodate your coping styles to help each of you get your needs met.

A Time to Tell, Not Show

Why is communication essential? The answer is simple: when we communicate, we can understand and be understood. The result: confusion over the impact infertility has had on you and your partner decreases; the more you understand each other, the more intimacy increases.

How do you communicate? That's more challenging. Some ways of communicating are less effective than others. Consider your doctor talking one hundred miles per hour about all the tests you need to have done—he's telling you so much so fast that it's hard, even overwhelming, to absorb what he's saying. Consider your three-year-old nephew throwing a tantrum—he's communicating, but it's hard to figure out how to soothe his frustration while he's screaming. When your husband withdraws into silence, he is communicating, but you must guess what he is trying to say—is he angry? Sad? Tired? Depressed? Just quiet? Since you can't read his mind, you are as likely to be wrong as right. Conversely, if your wife bursts into tears at the drop of a hat, she too is communicating—but what? Are they tears of anger? Tears of sadness? Tears from hormones? If she cannot put words to the tears, how can you help?

Communicating about infertility can be problematic since very often you yourself don't know exactly what you are feeling. It helps to pause in your most emotional moments and think about what you feel, rather than just *feel*. If you are in the midst of an argument, try, as a couple, to take a quick time-out (sufficiently brief that no one withdraws completely) to give each of you time to regroup. Reflecting gives you the choice of whether to express your anger directly to your partner, write it down, or talk to someone other than your partner. Putting an argument on "pause" gives you time to consider whether it should be pursued.

Despite the intense feelings that couples have, you really can help each other cope if you understand your partner's needs and feelings. This is a time to tell, not show. Words are one of your strongest tools in your effort to maintain intimacy and avoid alienation.

What do you say? How do you ask your partner to help if you don't know yourself? A good place to start is with the reproductive story. If you can tell your story to your partner, you are sharing your lost dreams. And you can hear your partner's lost dreams too. They may be similar, they may be different—but either way, the more you understand about each other, the tighter the emotional bond you share.

Time to Negotiate

When we say it's time to negotiate, we don't mean trying to get your partner to be the *same* as you. Once again, you and your partner should not expect to be clones of each other. Rather we mean that you find a way for *each of you* to cope as you need to without leaving the other feeling flattened or lost. Negotiation, though, is only possible once you have found the words to communicate what you need and how you can best obtain it.

Negotiation usually means a compromise is in order. When loss of control is so powerful, as it is with infertility, you may resist finding a middle ground, but we have found this helpful for many couples.

As you communicate and negotiate with your partner, remember that this process is a lengthy one—not everything is going to get sorted out right away. Always keep in mind that each of you is struggling to deal with your own reproductive story. If ever there was a time to give each other the benefit of the doubt, now is it. If you can translate your partner's behavior into feelings and words, or better yet, if you can ask your spouse to translate it for you, you will almost certainly find not a mean, cold, uncaring, overly emotional, demanding, or critical spouse, but someone who, like you, is in pain and needs help.

Finally, it is important to remember that you are not trapped or controlled by your partner. Your relationship isn't traumatic; the crisis of infertility is. Your partner is neither controlling you nor causing the awful feelings; instead, the bad feelings come from your thwarted efforts to become parents, and the circumstances— larger than either of you—have taken away your control.

If You Are Still Pulling Apart

Sometimes, though, if there is something wrong with the relationship, infertility makes it worse. Relationships crack along existing fault lines when something as earthshaking as infertility hits. A couple may unconsciously hope that having a baby together will correct the problems in their relationship. Then the stakes really go sky-high.

In many cases, the crisis of infertility can spur a couple to get the help they need as a couple. If you still find yourselves pushing apart, we recommend couples counseling to have a safe haven in which to try to work through your underlying conflicts, and then together work through the issues that are specific to the infertility.

Sometimes, however, a couple realizes that the primary problem in their lives is not infertility, but the relationship itself. They come to recognize that even if they could conceive, a baby could not heal the rifts or incompatibility between them.

Ultimately, you each have to decide whether to stay together or not. Sometimes it is harder to leave, sometimes it is harder to stay. But whichever way you go, let it be an informed choice, not an angry reaction.

Reconnecting

In spite of all the ways infertility can come between couples, we have found that many couples grow closer as a result. They counter the sense of isolation that they feel with their family or peers by sticking together. This "us against the world" bond is bolstered by their partner's support. And their infertility crisis heightens their awareness of how much they love and need each other.

Over the course of five years, Jeannie and Hank have been through surgeries, a miscarriage, and two failed IVF cycles. "We've had so many ups and downs," said Jeannie, "but through it all Hank has been wonderful. I feel closer to him than ever."

Hank agreed. "Through this we realized how much family means to both of us. Not just having kids, but our parents and siblings, and of course, each other. And we are going to have kids, one way or another."

Wherever you are in your journey, be aware of your partner's vulnerability. Remind each other that neither you nor your relationship has to be defined by infertility. We encourage couples to focus on the positive, healthy sides of their relationship whenever they can, while simultaneously pursuing treatment. Go on dates (with each other!) or take weekend trips; carving out special time helps renew what you enjoy about each other.

When you can take a break from treatment, even just a month here and there as long as medically permitted, use that time to regain a sense of your "old selves." You can reinforce the positive aspects of your connection, re-engage in spontaneous sex, and give both your bodies and minds time to rest, before moving on to the next intervention.

In the end, try to recognize that your reproductive selves are only a part of who you are—both individually and as a couple. You are in this together, for better or for worse, but there is more to the two of you. While the trauma of infertility may be all-consuming now, it's just one chapter in the story of your lives together.

PART III

Grieving and Coping

Eight

Grieving for the Pregnancy or the Baby that Never Was

This month I thought it finally happened. After four years of infertility, my period was three days late—and I'm never late. I actually imagined wrapping a cigar in pink-and-blue ribbons and presenting it to my husband. I was trying not to get excited, but the truth is I was ecstatic. It was finally my turn to have a baby! But the next day, when I went into the bathroom, there it was: that bright spot of hated red. Once again, no baby. How many more months can I go through these little deaths?

—Stacy, infertile four years

In this chapter, we explore the arduous task you face when mourning the "little deaths" Stacy refers to. So many people fail to understand that infertility elicits a kind of grief similar to the loss of a loved one, yet the grief of infertility is that much more challenging because there is no actual person to mourn. Having to grieve when a birth is anticipated is illogical; it's out of line with the normal and expected course of a life. There is a nothingness, an emptiness, that needs to be grieved in the same way as other losses. But how do you mourn a baby or a pregnancy that never was? How can you have a funeral for a longing or a wish? How do you mourn your own loss of identity as a parent? And how many times must you grieve the same kind of loss when month after month the cycle repeats itself?

Although it is not easy to grieve fully when there is a chance that next month, or with the next intervention, a successful pregnancy may occur, mourning the "little deaths" is very important; otherwise, grief can get stored up and cause more emotional problems later on.

The Complicated Task of Grieving Infertility
How Do We Mourn When No One Has Died?

As painful as it is to lose someone close to us, mourning that kind of loss is made easier by reminiscing about the person. Being able to recall the times spent with a family member or friend—shared meals, shopping outings, vacations, work, good times, and bad—all these fund a rich supply of memories that will never be erased. Sharing the account of the deceased's life with others enhances and aids the mourning process. Eulogies given at funerals celebrate and recognize the treasured memories and feelings that person has bestowed. As Leo recalled: "After my father died, my mother and sister and I sat at the dining room table with a stack of old photographs. We laughed, we cried, we spent hours remembering old times. It was helpful to know that he was still alive in our hearts."

But with infertility, there are no such memories to call upon for solace, no photographs, no chronicles of a life. Infertile couples know that what they're going through feels like a death in the family—and more. Not only must you grieve the absence of a baby—and the loss of the desired experience of pregnancy—you must also grieve the loss of your dreams, hopes, and expectations of having a family—in other words, your reproductive story. In addition, a piece of yourself is lost: that piece that you hold as a potential parent. Grieving still must take place, but in the absence of any concrete reminders, the mourning process is that much more difficult.

Because no actual person has died, it follows that there are no rituals—religious, cultural, or otherwise—to guide you through the reproductive grieving process. No funerals, wakes, headstones, or sitting shiva accompany the arrival of a period when a procedure has failed. In fact, there is a very good chance that the only people who know about the loss are you, your partner, and perhaps your doctor. Alone with your loss, you are forced to grieve with very little, if any, support. This is a very private, very devastating grief.

Even if couples do find support from their family and friends, they still complain that they feel alone. Stacy remarked with anger that people didn't understand the impact these "little deaths" were having on her. "If I told an acquaintance that my favorite uncle just passed away," she said, "I know I would get sympathy and understanding from them. They would be able to relate. But if I told them that my period arrived once again—they would look at me as if I were from another planet. Or else they might give me those horrid, encouraging words: 'Oh, you can always try again next month,' that only make me feel worse. On the outside, it appears that everything is the same, like nothing has happened, nothing has changed, and yet this is the saddest time of my life."

What Stacy knows only too well is that unless people have experienced infertility themselves, it can be very hard for them to relate to the extent of the pain and the depth of the loss that infertile couples face.

How Do We Grieve if We're Still Trying?

Added to the isolation and lack of support for couples, you may also feel as if you cannot fully grieve while you are still in the process of trying to have a baby. If you may possibly conceive next month, how can you get any sense of closure on the experience? You're living in a cycle of hope (during ovulation) followed by the enormous letdown (when conception doesn't take place) followed by hope once again. This pattern, which often lasts for years, makes it seem impossible to fully resolve the loss.

It's similar to a boxer in the ring who is losing the match, but is determined to keep going. He gets knocked down, gets up, only to get knocked down again. And with each round he gets a little more hurt, a little more disorientated, a little less able to regroup—but still hopeful of a win, he remains in the ring. When the bell rings marking the end of the match, he can nurse his wounds and recuperate. But when does the final bell ring for infertile couples?

If you are still in the ring, it is very difficult to grieve each month. With the thread of hope, however thin, dangling in front of you, the task of grieving may seem unnecessary or too final. Each month it may feel as if you are getting one step closer to the end of the road and the desire to deny this is normal. You may feel you are giving up the fight if you let yourself grieve, and so the wish to disavow the feelings or blame them on something else may take over. It is essential, however, to face the grief even as you continue to pursue treatment. Acknowledging the multiple losses from month to month will not eliminate your pain, but releasing the pent-up feelings of anger, frustration, and sadness will provide some relief.

Even when couples have decided to move on, a persistent, niggling ounce of hope may remain that maybe—just maybe—a pregnancy still might happen. Elena and her husband, Ray, have stopped seeing their infertility specialist and agreed that they need to pursue other avenues toward parenthood. Nevertheless, Elena, who has just celebrated her forty-sixth birthday, is, unbeknownst to Ray, still trying to conceive. "The rational side of me knows that having a biological child at this point in my life is next to impossible. But I am still menstruating regularly, I know exactly when I ovulate, and I make sure we have sex during that time. And each month, I secretly hope my actions will pay off. It seems crazy that I am still pursuing this, but I can't help myself."

Elena's sense of hope keeps the door open, but it also may get in the way of her having some closure on this phase of her life. She does not want to admit defeat, even though she knows it's a losing battle. It is perfectly normal and reasonable to hold onto hope, even if the odds are against you. We have experienced it ourselves, and have seen it time and again with our clients—the feeling that having a baby, no matter what any doctor has said, still just might happen. Yet holding onto false hope, as natural as it is, may interfere with your ability to make decisions about your future. It may hamper you from moving on to the next chapter in your life.

So How Do We Get Through This?

What we have found as therapists, and in our own personal experience, is that while it's absolutely necessary to grieve so you can heal from infertility's wounds, the roadblocks to honoring this grief are many. The first step is to recognize and realize that what you are going through is real. Even though others may not see your loss as comparable to a death in the family, it truly is. Infertility causes genuine loss—really multiple losses as we have seen—that needs to be mourned just like the loss of any loved one.

The second step is to understand just how difficult mourning infertility can be. Remember that you are dealing with an intangible loss, one that is private and one that few understand. You're also grieving the loss of hope—having a baby—while at the same time trying to remain hopeful for your next attempt.

The third step is to become familiar with the phases typical of the grief process. Knowing the challenges of mourning up front can be reassuring, as illustrated in the next section.

What is Grief?

Grief is an intense emotional reaction to a loss. The loss, real or threatened, can be of anything to which you are strongly attached. It is not merely sadness, but a response felt throughout your body. It can affect your physical well-being, causing discomforts such as breathing problems, muscle aches, gastrointestinal pain, or exhaustion. Grief can affect your behavior: some people throw themselves into work, others into alcohol or drugs; some can't sleep, while others may take naps as an escape. Likewise, your eating habits may change, and you might gain or lose weight. You'll feel sad, but you may also feel angry, confused, frightened, or helpless. And grief can also wreak havoc on your sense of self as you come to terms with guilt and regret about things you may have done in the past.

Renee, a thirty-four-year-old teacher, entered therapy after being diagnosed with endometriosis. She had gone for a routine checkup after a year of unsuccessful trying, only to get news she hadn't expected. Now, six months after her diagnosis, she was still shaken and wondering why this had happened to her. Day-to-day living had become a grind, and her husband had become impatient with her despondent and angry moods.

"Phil is sick and tired of me. He was understanding and sympathetic at first. He even came with me to my doctor's appointments. But now, truth be told, he avoids me like the plague. I think the remote control has become his best friend. If I get weepy or complain, he shuts down. He says he's sick of hearing about not having children. Of course, he has been upset about it too. But his feeling is you get over it, and you go on. But I can't seem to do that. I don't know what I am supposed to do. Pretend I'm okay? Pretend it doesn't hurt? I need to talk to him, but he doesn't want to hear it anymore."

As her story unfolded, it became clear that the distance between Phil and Renee was a result not just of their infertility trauma, but also how they coped with their grief. We have found that men and women tend to grieve differently, especially in the face of infertility. It is easier for women to cry openly when they are sad; it is culturally more acceptable for women to voice their feelings. Men, however, often feel that they need to be the cheerleader, keep a stiff upper lip, and channel their grief into support for their partner, as we discussed in chapter 6.

Ernie and his wife, Mara, have been through eight years of infertility treatment, including six IUIs and two failed IVF procedures. They are currently investigating an egg-donor program as well as adoption. Ernie said, "I know we will get to be parents somehow. I am positive about that." In private, however, Ernie confided that he often goes for long drives "so I can be alone in the car and cry." He couldn't show his vulnerable side to Mara because he thought he needed to be strong for her. He was also afraid he would upset her more if she knew how upset he sometimes was.

Not only do men and women often grieve differently, people also grieve in different ways and at different times. Phil viewed grieving as a condition, like having a cold or the flu. You feel lousy for a while, stay in bed, and nurse yourself back to health, but then the symptoms abate, and you return to your former level of functioning. But for most people, grieving doesn't happen in a straight uphill line—from feeling bad to getting well again. Instead, it's like a wave that ebbs and flows, ebbs and flows.

And each time you revisit or relive a loss, you view and handle it differently as time goes on. It's like rereading a book: you get something else out of every reading. As we discuss in the next sections, there are different components and phases of grief; each time you re-enter a phase, your outlook slightly alters. Usually with time and distance from the particular loss, symptoms lessen. But grieving infertility is particularly difficult because you can't gain distance if the loss repeats itself month after month.

The Stages of Grief

Most research on mourning points to a series of stages that people go through, from initial shock and denial, to feelings of sadness, anger, and self-blame, then the hope for a miracle, and finally, acceptance. Although these stages are listed in a certain order, implying that you pass through one phase, complete it, and move on to the next, the truth is that grieving infertility is *not* a linear process. You may experience these stages simultaneously or in a jumbled order over the course of months or years. One morning, you may accept your infertility, yet later that afternoon you may feel full of rage. These unpredictable emotions are normal; they do not mean you are losing your mind, or that you're failing at grieving on top of everything else you have gone through.

This Can't be Happening to Me!

Denial and shock are two of the most common characteristics of initial grieving. No one wants to believe awful news. When the news is of a personal nature—when your doctor tells you that you have endometriosis or poor sperm quality, and that your chances of getting pregnant are greatly reduced—the shock is particularly overwhelming. We hear from our patients all the time: "I can't believe it! This just can't be happening to *me!*"

Renee described the appointment when her doctor first suspected that something was wrong with her reproductive system. "My periods had been painful with more intense cramps than usual, but I chalked it up to PMS. When I mentioned it to my doctor at my routine appointment—the cramping and trying to get pregnant for a year—he ordered more tests," she said. "I could feel myself tuning out as he listed what could be causing me problems. I kept thinking that he had to be wrong—nothing was the matter with me, it was just cramps. I honestly don't remember hearing half of what he said as he quoted percentages and procedures. All I remember is wanting him to stop talking so I could go home and crawl under the blankets."

Renee, caught completely off guard, went into shock—a normal reaction to getting unexpected bad news. Also normal was her desire to shut out the world and deny the reality of painful information.

"Phil was in shock too," she continued. "That night when I told him, we both just sat and stared at our dinner, barely able to eat. Phil suggested we schedule another appointment with my doctor so he could come and ask questions. I was grateful for that."

What helped Renee, like most people when they first receive an infertility diagnosis, was to compile as much information as possible and not feel alone in what was happening. We recommend taking another person with you to your appointments; it helps you first to take in what your doctor is saying and later to make what may be some difficult decisions.

In addition, being able to voice your thoughts, concerns, sadness, and fears with your partner can help you come out from under the covers, lessen the need for denial, and face the reality of the situation. When you are able to talk about your feelings, they become less burdensome. Things become unspeakable and overwhelming when they are kept inside; when you give voice to them, they become more manageable and less frightening.

One Minute I'm Crying, the Next I'm in a Rage

When the reality of the situation sinks in, you may feel sad and depressed, angry and frustrated, and anxious and pessimistic about the future. All these emotions can occur at once and overwhelm you, but these are all normal reactions when the reproductive story does not go as planned, and all a normal part of the grief process.

You may feel despondent and hopeless, heartbroken and down in the dumps. Felice, a thirty-nine-year-old attorney, had been di-

agnosed with age-related infertility. Although her doctor was optimistic about her chances of getting pregnant using ART or donor
technology, Felice did not feel the same way. "It's hard to want to
pursue the list of options the doctor gave me," she said. "I feel like
giving up before I even get started."

Intertwined with her despair were feelings of intense anger. Although the power of these emotions can be unnerving, they are a
normal component of grief. Felice felt most angry with herself for
delaying childbearing. "I was always waiting for the right time to
have kids, but it never seemed convenient. I always found an excuse for waiting," she said. "If I hadn't put it off, I wouldn't be in
this mess. I could kick myself for waiting as long as I did."

Renee, too, admonished herself. "Why didn't I go see the doctor when I first had signs of pain? Now, looking back, I know I was
in denial. I wanted to believe that nothing was wrong."

Anger in the mourning process gets directed outward as well.
You may find yourself more irritable with your partner, or with
anyone who crosses your path who happens to have a child. Often
it's the people we are closest to who bear the brunt of our emotional eruptions. It's not because we suddenly see all their faults
and discover that we hate them; it's the opposite. We can let out
our anger with the people we are closest to because they are safe:
they will love us no matter what. But at the same time it can be
confusing to explode at the people you love—and after doing so
you may feel more hurt and upset, and scared that your intimate
relationships are falling apart.

We advise clients to remember that the infertility and grief fuel
the anger. Your relationships are not falling apart because of some
fatal flaw in you or in them; rather, it's the trauma and loss you are

experiencing that's wreaking havoc on your sense of self and on your relationships. Realizing that this is a normal and expected grief reaction can help you better prepare for this emotional roller coaster.

How can you release these emotions constructively? Renee utilized therapy to put her sadness and anger into perspective. Talking about her feelings helped her understand why mourning is necessary and that anger is a natural part of that mourning.

Vigorous exercise can also alleviate tension and stress. Physical activity releases endorphins, which help reduce pain and promote a sense of well-being. In addition, writing, drawing, or other creative activities can feel cathartic and bring relief. When Diana, infertile for five years, found out that her third IVF had failed, she was driving home, listening to a Beethoven symphony. "The music flooded me. I had to stop driving to listen. I was crying so hard—tears of sadness and tears of rage poured out of me. I pounded on the steering wheel, I was so angry. If anyone saw me, I can't imagine what they thought was going on. Afterward, though, I felt a lot better. It was like a weight had lifted off of me. It felt like I had somehow been purged."

It requires immense energy to hold in our feelings; letting them out, as Diana described, can feel liberating. Letting go of them in a manner that doesn't point the finger at yourself or others is especially beneficial.

Remember that infertility creates a state of chronic and repeated trauma. You may want to control your emotions to help feel more in control of your life, but discharging your feelings will actually make you feel better. Sometimes you may not even recognize the connection between these intense emotions and the trauma of infertility. When sadness or anger overtakes you suddenly, it is often difficult to remember that this is a crucial element of mourning. But it is essential to release these feelings, so vital emotional energy isn't continually used up to stuff them in. The danger is in getting stuck—denying these feelings—which masks your sadness or anger. It's as if your backpack of emotions gets heavier and heavier, which leads to more depressed feelings and more anxiety.

If I Wish Upon a Star, Will My Dreams Come True?

Who can forget Jiminy Cricket crooning, *"When you wish upon a star . . . "* in Disney's classic, *Pinocchio.* The only way poor old Geppetto was going to get a *real* boy was to rely on the good graces of the Blue Fairy. If only we had a fairy at our beck and call to make all our reproductive wishes come true.

Lacking a fairy godmother, a magic wand, or other such charms, what we do have to hold on to in the midst of our anguish over infertility is hope. Hope provides us with the strength to persevere. Hoping for our dream to come true, wishing for a miracle—these feelings are not rational or logical. Nonetheless, these feelings exist without our even being aware of it. And just like the emotions of sadness and anger, hoping for a miracle is an integral part of grieving.

Negotiating deals, making promises, setting up scenarios where you will be able to have a baby *if* you act accordingly—these, too, are all part of the grief process. Many an infertile couple find themselves pleading for a chance at having a baby. "I would do *anything* to have a baby," so many of our clients tell us. In desperation, people often try to change and perfect their own behavior, as if that makes the difference between having a baby and not. Holly, whose doctors haven't been able to find a conclusive source of her infertility, listed her "faults," which included:

- not exercising enough
- not flossing every day
- not calling her family enough
- paying bills late
- eating too many sweets
- watching too much TV

"When I look over this list," she said, "it doesn't make any sense that these things would prevent me from having a baby. Rationally I understand all this. But another part of me feels like if I promise to do better—to take better care of myself and my things and the people around me—then I'll deserve a baby and only then will it happen."

Many infertility patients try one intervention after another; afraid to stop the process, they always hope that if they make the right bargain, come upon the right formula, then this time it will work. When Elena secretly tries to conceive, even though she knows the odds are against her, she is hoping for a miracle. In our magical thinking, we believe that if we behave in the right way, we will have a positive outcome. It's like hoping for Santa to bring a much wished-for bicycle—we try our best to be good boys or girls, hoping that our good behavior will be recognized and rewarded with a baby. The reasonable and logical parts of our thinking know that these behaviors are not at all connected, but irrational thoughts tend to creep in when we are feeling vulnerable and desperate for explanations.

When we feel as if there is nothing else we can do, we pray, we hope, we wish, and we make private deals with ourselves in order to insure that what we want will come our way. It buoys us up at a time of despair and is yet another stage of the grief process.

Resolution

Most of the literature on death and dying posits that after going through all the other phases of grief—the shock, the sadness, the anger, the hope, and bargaining—you will come to the point of resolution. No longer in turmoil over the loss, it is said, you can move forward, find peace and acceptance. Although this may hold true for many situations, infertility is uniquely different. Infertility is not a single loss, but consists of multiple layers of loss. And there isn't always a definitive end. For some couples, only after the birth (or adoption) of their child do they feel resolution. Others feel, however, that resolution is still not possible even after the birth of a child. More on this point will be discussed in chapter 12, but suffice it to say that infertility is a life-altering event, which we must learn to cope with and incorporate into our reproductive story.

Full resolution implies that you have come to a firm conclusion about infertility. But if you are still in the midst of trying, such final resolution is not possible. Additional failures increase the sense of loss and make the grieving process that much more difficult. When each month brings another defeat, you will not have enough time to grieve that loss before you get your hopes up again for the next try. Each loss along the way reopens the wound that you are trying to heal.

Not only do couples grieve each month, they also grieve when they shift from one reproductive technique to another. Each change in the technology you choose may feel like another loss. Going from "the old-fashioned way" to using any number of ART procedures can feel like a defeat. Likewise, deciding to forgo your own genetic child and use donor egg or sperm, or to adopt instead, may be exciting, but may also feel like a failure and a new loss.

Because of Renee's endometriosis, she and Phil decided to pursue a gestational surrogate. To arrive at this decision, Renee had to grieve the loss of experiencing pregnancy. She described her acceptance: "Each step along the way brought me further and further away from my original reproductive story. It finally sunk in that I wasn't going to have a baby as I had originally thought I would. And as it sunk in, I guess you could say that I became open to other ways to become a mom. But this hasn't been easy."

This "sinking in," as Renee called it, is really the process of resolution. An important distinction should be made here—the difference between *resolution* and *resignation*. Resolution means you have come to a firm and clear decision—in Renee's case, using a surrogate. Resignation, however, is giving in because you feel you have no other options. In coping with infertility, the difference between resolution and resignation is vast. It can mean the difference between accepting the necessary changes to your reproductive story or feeling as if you are stuck; or between fully integrating a new ending to your reproductive story or continuing to experience turmoil and despair.

You may be able to accept a new ending to your story today, but feel unsure of it tomorrow. These vacillations, too, are normal. Once again, the phases of grief are not linear; people move in and out of them, only to repeat them again and again. It may feel frustrating to think that a phase has been finished and then land in the midst of it again. Each time through the feelings, however, provides a new outlook and perspective, ultimately bringing you closer to a sense of resolution.

The "Little Deaths"

The "little deaths" that you experience can and should be mourned, but often they are overlooked by family, friends, the medical community, and sometimes even by ourselves as we're undergoing treatment.

After struggling with infertility for four years, Suzanne came in one day beaming. "I have something to show you!" In her hand was a picture from her IVF procedure, and she pointed with pride to the embryos in the photo. "It's the first picture for our baby album!"

A week later, Suzanne was grief-stricken. The embryos failed to implant, and, according to her doctors, this was not considered a pregnancy at all. Technically speaking, the doctors were right; this really wasn't a bona fide pregnancy. But for Suzanne, it *had* been a pregnancy. The picture she brought in had been of her baby. "But I *was* pregnant," she cried. "For a moment, I really *felt* pregnant. And now it's gone."

As Suzanne noted, even though she was not *officially* pregnant, she *felt* pregnant. In part, this happens because medical technology allowed her to experience, both visually and emotionally, a process of human development that most people never see. For

Suzanne, feeling pregnant and losing the pregnancy all occurred before most women even have a clue that they have conceived. The loss of her pregnancy was as real to her as any other loss might be.

These "pregnant moments" described by Suzanne need to be incorporated into the grieving process. When in vitro fertilization has occurred, infertile couples often experience the embryos as potential babies and find themselves already feeling emotionally attached. When those cells don't implant, couples feel as if a baby has been taken from them. Until recently, there has not even been a name for such a "death," which some researchers are now calling a "pre-implantation miscarriage," or "non-carriage." Giving this loss a label makes it that much more real, allowing couples to feel validated in their grief.

A failed IVF, however, is not the same as a miscarriage. Having a confirmed pregnancy after going through infertility carries with it a confirmation that you can conceive. Such validation is missing if an IVF doesn't take, or resolves as a chemical pregnancy. But even with a miscarriage, couples often feel alone and misunderstood, as if this, too, were a nonevent. Well-meaning but insensitive remarks from friends and family (such as "it wasn't meant to be" or "you can always try again") only add to the couples' anguish.

Eva suffered a miscarriage at eight weeks after three years of infertility treatment. "My sister-in-law said, 'You're lucky. At least it was early.'" Eva was furious with her sister-in-law for discounting her feelings. "I wanted to scream at her, 'What if your daughter was in a car accident and died? How would you feel then? Because that's how I feel now.'"

Rituals for the "Little Deaths"

One major problem in dealing with this kind of loss—be it a miscarriage, chemical pregnancy, non-carriage, or the monthly period—is that no commonly accepted rituals exist to help guide you or your loved ones through the grief. We believe, however, that having a ritual helps to acknowledge these intangible and very private losses. It is not for others that a ritual is necessary, although it may also aid those close to you who are looking for a way to help. The ritual is for you and your partner, to allow you to validate the reality of your pain and loss.

One ritual we suggest is for couples to set aside a special time either weekly or monthly. Sophie and her husband, Tom, go out for dinner once a month when Sophie's period arrives, no matter what day of the week and no matter what else they may have had scheduled. What may at first glance seem like a celebration is not. Their dinner date allows them to spend time together, and acknowledge yet another sad moment in their journey. Sophie admitted that many times she feels so low that she doesn't want to go. "But ultimately I am glad I do," she said. "It always makes me feel that I am not in this alone. It forces us to talk. Lots of times we don't even bring up the baby issue. I think if we didn't do this each month, I would close up—this forces me to work on us even when I don't feel like it."

From Tom's perspective he treasures these dinners. "My work would eat me up if I let it. It's easier for me to avoid emotional things than to deal with them," he said. "That's why having this time with Sophie has been so good for our relationship. I just wish we could be celebrating instead. But in a way it forces us to take stock of what we *do* have, rather than only focus on what we don't."

Other rituals we recommend for couples to acknowledge their monthly loss include going for a walk together, lighting a candle, or buying each other a flower. If you have had a miscarriage or a failed IVF, you may want to memorialize this event in a more substantial way. Molly, who miscarried after an IVF procedure, planted a tree in her backyard. "I had been feeling so helpless after the miscarriage that it made me feel better to do something—but especially something positive. It felt good to plant a sapling that I could nurture and watch grow. It helps to have this visual reminder that I *was* pregnant and that for that short time I was the best mother I could possibly be."

Other couples have chosen to mark the date on their calendars and, each year on the anniversary, find a way to commemorate the loss. Often anniversaries of the loss, or the baby's expected due date, can be just as distressing as the actual loss. Many of our clients comment that they feel sad, irritable, or unwell, seemingly for no reason, on or around the calendar date of their loss. Because these grief reactions seem to come out of the blue, knowing that they are normal and to be anticipated can help save us from feeling bowled over by them.

Yet another potentially helpful ritual is more public than private. Perhaps you can organize or become involved in a walk for individuals and couples who have experienced reproductive trauma and loss. Or you can attend a workshop on infertility or reproductive loss. Participating in these kinds of events, or even helping develop them, is another way to establish a ritual to help you grieve.

Many of our clients have described the solace they have found in doing *something*. No matter what it is that you decide to do, this loss needs to be recognized and not hidden in some out-of-reach place. Creating a ritual for the pregnancy or baby that never was can help you make real that which has been so intangible.

Getting Stuck in Grief

Inevitably, in the course of grieving a reproductive trauma, you will have moments when you feel stuck—either in a mood, a phase of grief, or obsessive rumination. Ilene was so distraught that she literally got stuck on her sofa. She found herself blankly staring out the window, and when she finally looked up, she discovered that over an hour had passed. Having structure—something to do—can be a way out of these terribly despondent times. Sometimes mustering up the energy to do something feels like it is just too much, but having a focus or task, like going to work, or attending a support group, exercise class, or other activity can help get you through it.

Even the most well-meaning people often imply that you should be "over it" and able to "get on with life." This can make you feel even worse—not only are you struggling with infertility, you may feel as though you are not even grieving right. Patients who have been encouraged to talk about their infertility sometimes get the impression that they have talked about it *too* much. Nina, infertile for three years, feels as if she has alienated and "used up" her support network. "I think my friends are sick of me and my problems. I try not to dwell on my treatment, but I really do need to talk about it. If I can't talk to them, who else is there?"

Phoebe has similar concerns. "My mother is avoiding me; I know it. I know it's hard for her to see me in pain, but what am I supposed to do? Whenever I've tried to talk to her about my infertility she has this unnerving way of changing the subject. I wind up feeling like I have to take care of her—that she's the one suffering here—and not me. I get the feeling from her that I should just forget about it all and move on."

Especially painful are the times when you and your partner are at different points in the grieving process. A very common scenario is that he has "put it behind him," wants to move forward, and can't understand why she is still feeling so devastated. And she can't understand how he could be so insensitive and not recognize the giant emptiness inside her! At times like these, you may feel as if you are doing everything wrong. Knowing that people grieve in their own ways and that you and your partner may experience these losses differently can help you understand each other at this crucial and sensitive time. You don't want to let the differences in your individual grieving styles and timetables cripple the relationship.

When you get the message—from your partner, friends, or family—that you should be "over" this, it not only makes you feel misunderstood, it also adds to the feeling that you are all alone. If you feel as if you have used up your resources—your friends and family—you may want to consider joining a support group (see the resource section in the back of the book) and/or pursue psychotherapy or counseling.

Support groups can be lifesavers. Hearing others discuss their plight and talking about your own actually helps facilitate grieving.

Getting to know other people who are going through a similar experience can ease the pain of isolation. Gillian found her support group so helpful that she eventually became a member of the board. "I knew I could talk about my feelings, and someone in the group would understand. I never felt like I was overloading others with my problems—we were all in it together."

Therapy, either individually or as a couple, can also help the grief process. Setting aside time each week to talk with a therapist can provide enormous relief. Knowing there is a time and place to "unload" can be a source of great comfort and solace. Being able to bring your feelings into therapy and leave them there each session has the added benefit of freeing you from carrying the burden all by yourself. Many of our psychotherapy clients sigh with relief knowing that, "My session is tomorrow. I get time to talk!" It can be freeing to know that your thoughts and feelings will be acknowledged without being judged or burdening someone else.

We have seen many couples enter therapy so angry that they could barely talk to one another. Evan and Liza began therapy because they were arguing all the time. Whenever they had tried talking things out at home, they ended up in a blowout. To avoid these painful combative duels, Evan began spending more and more time at work, which infuriated Liza even more. The more he avoided her, the more nagging she became; he'd storm out of the house and the pattern continued.

They were able to break this cycle in therapy as they realized the strength of their relationship. Liza said, "Talking about our relationship in therapy, I began to appreciate Evan all over again. He really is a great guy. We have so much in common. I now understand that he's been in as much pain as I have."

Evan concurred. "We really have the same goals. We both want a family so much; I know Liza will be a great mother. Neither one of us knew what to do with our frustration. We took it out on each other."

Utilizing couples therapy, Liza and Evan were able to separate their struggles with infertility from the rest of their relationship. Therapy helped them to see that their anger toward each other was really part of their grief—grief that their reproductive story and dreams of a family were not to be as they had hoped. As they faced their grief together, they were able to mend and heal, as individuals and as a couple, and come to an agreement about the next step in treatment.

How to Get "Unstuck"

As we have learned, grieving infertility is a long and arduous process. Unlike a predictable bus or train schedule, you and your partner will each have your own timetable for grief. What makes grieving these "little deaths" so much more complicated is that you are still in the *middle* of your reproductive story—not at the beginning and not at the end. In fact, the prolonged nature of infertility makes resolving grief very difficult. You are forced to grieve the same loss over and over each time it occurs.

So what helps? First and foremost, it is essential to communicate. Talk about your feelings with your partner, friends, family, and your therapist. Even though Renee wanted to "crawl under the blankets" when she found out about her endometriosis, she didn't. She talked with Phil and garnered his support. If talking isn't possible, write down your feelings. Creating your infertility diary is a great way to release your feelings. Any way you can get the feelings from inside of you to outside will help. This gives you the chance to reflect on your feelings, rather than feeling overwhelmed and controlled by them. Admit when you feel upset. Denying your feelings and bottling them up is more destructive in the long run. It takes far more courage to acknowledge your emotional pain openly than to ignore it.

Along with this, try to find ways to vent the anger that accompanies grief. If you have a friend or therapist who understands your situation, go ahead and rail in outrage at the insensitive remarks others sometimes make. Sarcastic humor, used in the right context, can be a valuable tool for venting if it comes naturally to you. Molly laughed and cried at the list of stinging retorts she and her close friend, Becky, composed after Molly's miscarriage. "We just let it rip! I didn't know I could be so nasty!" Molly said. "Here's my favorite: someone says, 'Have you considered adoption?'—my retort—'I'd seriously think about it if I looked like you!' It's not that I'd ever use any of these, but saying them secretly to myself actually helps. But what helped the most was spending the afternoon with Becky and letting it all out." Becky's coaxing and support gave Molly permission to get "unstuck" from her anger.

Be true to yourself. Don't try to feel a certain way because someone else thinks you should. It's okay not to feel grateful if someone tries to cheer you by saying, "you can keep trying" or "you can always adopt" or any number of other well-meaning remarks. As much as it helps to talk about infertility, it's also okay not to talk about it if you are not in the mood. Being tuned in to your own needs allows you to be kind to yourself and your partner.

Even if you get frustrated at times, be patient with yourself.

Holly's list of her "faults" allowed her to separate infertility from the rest of herself. She could then grieve her loss rather than focus on herself as a bad person. Likewise, be patient with your partner. Treat each other with the utmost kindness. Like Sophie and Tom's monthly dinner date, creating time to spend with each other away from the grind and chores of daily living can help you stay connected. The tenderness that you would expect to have for your much-wanted child needs to be transferred to your partner—and to yourself as well.

Above all, remember there is no right or wrong way to feel, no right or wrong way to manage all you have been through and continue to experience. It takes time to grieve. But just as Renee and Phil came to grips with her endometriosis and the necessary changes to their reproductive story, so will you. As Renee said, she needed to let things sink in before she could move forward with an alternate way to become a parent. You can't erase what you have been through but you can and will get through this, and this chapter of your reproductive story, albeit rewritten, will come to a close.

Nine

Dealing with the World

It's amazing, when you're experiencing infertility, how many times a day you are bombarded with "baby stuff." Is it our imagination, or do babies and pregnant women jump out at us everywhere? Are there suddenly more ads on TV for diapers? You may never have noticed so many pregnant bellies or baby strollers before, but now your sensitivity is heightened. Hearing a baby cry, seeing a neighbor with her kids, watching a stroller brigade march down the street—these daily reminders of the pain of infertility confront you wherever you turn.

It also may seem that whenever you get bad news—such as you're not pregnant again—someone else is celebrating good news. When a friend announces her pregnancy or a work colleague takes maternity leave, you may feel even more like the perennial odd woman or man out. While happy for your friend, you may feel more sad and sorry for yourself.

Conversations with close friends and family members can feel treacherous. You're always on guard against insensitive remarks or well-meaning but misguided advice. Even strangers who casually inquire when you're going to have kids can rub you wrong on an off day. You may feel incredibly angry and vulnerable.

If people haven't experienced infertility, they are not aware of how "in our face" it is almost every moment of every day. And they don't realize how much it can hurt.

Short of moving to a deserted island, you can't do anything to change the family-centric world we live in. We know how stressful it can be as you deal with the world of children, pregnant women, and advice-givers. In this chapter, we share coping strategies to help you handle the onslaught of infertility-insensitive situations you may face, such as:

- soothing yourself with self-talk when everyday situations leave you feeling hurt
- handling well-meaning but insensitive remarks from friends and family
- dealing with your family, from asking for their emotional support to possible financial help
- realizing it's perfectly okay *not* to attend family gatherings, parties, or baby showers if you're unsure about your ability to cope
- seeking outside support when you feel you need it

You Can Only Protect Yourself So Much

Usually we try to protect ourselves from situations that we think might cause us pain. Afraid someone is going to hurt you with an insensitive remark, you may find yourself avoiding friends or dodging conversations. You worry ahead of time about an offhand remark that can be cutting, and you do what you can to be on your guard.

But often it's the unanticipated situation that knocks us off our feet. Kathleen, on her way to a consult with a new infertility specialist for a second opinion, was already nervous going to his office located in the local hospital. As she recalled, "I became really unglued because his office was on the same floor as labor and delivery! Can you believe it? Even going to an infertility doctor I had to 'see' what I don't have."

The innocuous comments of strangers are also unwelcome. When Warren and Lila looked at the Labrador retriever puppies at a local pet store, the salesperson chatted them up. "Oh," he said, "aren't these puppies cute? These are the best dogs for kids. You two have kids?" Smiling and shaking their heads no, the couple quickly left the store, upset by this unexpected reminder of their childlessness.

Sometimes seeing mothers with babies can trigger unwelcome feelings too. Barbara became furious when she saw a mother ignoring her crying toddler in the supermarket. "I'm sure she's a good mom, but I can't stop myself from feeling that if I were given the chance, my baby wouldn't be crying like that," she said.

It's not easy to own up to the myriad feelings of sadness, inadequacy, anger, self-pity, and envy that can surface in everyday situations. But remember, you are experiencing trauma, with heightened feelings and reactions. So before you beat yourself up for feeling the way you do, acknowledge that those feelings are normal and understandable.

Self-Talk Can Save You

We have yet to meet an infertile couple who hasn't been zapped at one time or another by an everyday, unanticipated event. To survive these situations, we suggest a technique called *self-talk,* where you engage in an internal dialogue to boost your self-esteem. First, remind yourself that it's natural to have the feelings that you do. Of course you would be angry with your mother if she talked on and on about your sister's new baby; who wouldn't feel devastated if a forty-two-year-old friend announced her unplanned third pregnancy; and how could you not feel embarrassed to tell yet another person, "No, I don't have any kids"? Validating your own feelings is powerful, as you accept that you're reacting to a painful situation in a way that is to be expected.

But self-talk does more than validate your feelings about infertility. Self-talk allows you to think about yourself differently. When you feel bad, you can remind yourself over and over—like a broken record—of all that you do have going for you. Consider your intelligence, wit, talents, and skills. Thinking about your strengths while feeling devastated may seem easier said than done, but with practice, you'll find that you can pull yourself out of a rough spot rather quickly.

Monique, an advertising executive, utilized positive self-talk when she felt uncomfortable in a recreational cooking class. "When the instructor asked us to introduce ourselves, the first woman said she was a biologist and she had two kids. Next was the stay-at-home mom with four kids, a teacher with two kids, the next person had three. Out of ten women, I was the only one without children. When it was my turn, my heart was pounding so hard; I didn't know what to do."

Monique felt trapped—trapped by the situation and trapped by her infertility. Her impulse was to run out of the room. But instead, she began a dialogue with herself. *Okay,* she thought, *right now I feel completely out of place. All these other women seem like they've got it all, and I don't. But that's only because they have kids and I don't. At least not yet. Here's what I do have: I'm attractive, athletic, smart . . . I've got a job that I am good at, a wonderful husband who is my best friend . . . and I'm being creative by learning how to make desserts tonight.*

Talking to herself about her strengths and achievements, Monique remembered that having a child was only part of who she was. Regaining her composure, she introduced herself. By evening's end, not only did she learn some baking techniques, she had also exchanged phone numbers with several fellow bakers.

We help our clients learn to engage in this kind of active internal dialogue. Emphasizing the positive may seem hokey, but it works—you focus on what you *do* have, rather than on what is missing. Again, we want to emphasize how important is it to keep your infertility in perspective by placing it in the larger context of your life. Not only can self-talk can help you through some emotionally tough situations, it also gives you time to regroup whenever you feel down on yourself.

Responding to Stinging Remarks

Despite the efforts you make to protect yourself—especially by avoiding situations that you know will be particularly difficult (more on this later)—there invariably will be times when you are caught in unavoidable conversations. Most people don't mean to hurt you or to be insensitive, but sometimes they unwittingly are. Monique felt stung by all her cooking class companions announcing how many children they had. Of course those remarks weren't meant to be barbs, but they hurt nonetheless.

Infertile couples are asked all the time about having children, just as the pet store clerk asked Warren and Lila. The "Do you have kids?" question may be innocently posed, yet it can feel invasive and hurtful. It helps to remember why it feels so pointed—the question may tap into the shame and despair that you already feel about your inability to get pregnant.

To handle these situations, we suggest you brainstorm ahead of time how to respond to unwanted advice or well-meaning-but-invasive comments. This way, you are not taken by surprise and have a ready answer at hand. Answers like "not yet" or "soon" or "we're working on it" all work well—these brief responses are to the point and end the conversation.

Part of the problem with such questions is that you, like many people, feel that your reproductive life is private. Elaine, who decided to remain childfree after struggling with infertility, felt angry when people asked if she had children, but also thought she was being rude if she did not reply. Sometimes a humorous retort can ease the tension: "Not last time I checked" or "Yes, but they're invisible" might, at times, be appropriate. If your questioner persists and wants details that you are uncomfortable giving, be more direct by stating: "That's between my husband and me."

If someone knows you have had difficulty conceiving, they often make a clumsy attempt to console you. "Oh, be glad you don't have kids—I have four and they drive me crazy!" may be intended as comforting, but instead feels competitive and cruel. You may be tempted to retort, "Too bad you don't appreciate them. I know I would," or you may explain why you would love to have kids to drive you crazy.

Others feel remarkably free to give out advice on what to do. "Just relax—once you stop worrying about it, you'll get pregnant right away. That's what happened to my sister!" is another so-called helpful comment that too many people offer. But this comment is grossly insensitive, implying that your infertility is in your head and that somehow you are responsible for it. If you have a definite diagnosis, you may wish to share it; for example, you could explain how blocked tubes prevent conception from happening naturally, so there's nothing to relax about. You may also choose to educate the speaker, noting that infertility is a disease. Or you may just want to let them know how hurtful their "help" feels.

"My brother and his wife adopted a baby—and boom, she got pregnant" falls in the same category. You can say, "Yes, sometimes that happens, but did you ever think how many couples adopt and then don't get pregnant?" Or the offhand comment that, "Oh dear, my husband just has to look at me and I get pregnant" may be someone's effort to empathize but is incredibly thoughtless.

When you hear comments like these, remember that you do not have to respond right away, if at all. Focus on the person's conscious wish to be kind—most likely they feel awkward and don't know what to say—while you smile and count to five. That gives you time to choose a response. "Yes, that works for some people" or "It's different for everyone" is polite but reinforces the idea that your experience is different from theirs. Or these comments may make you want to lash out in anger. The desire to tell someone off is natural and you may be tempted to do so at times, but it's also an option to *not* respond when you feel the need for privacy. "I prefer to not talk about that right now," gets the message across loud and clear.

If you don't want to respond directly to the person who hurts you or makes you angry, it can be helpful to vent your feelings after the fact. A sarcastic retelling of the story to someone who really does understand how you feel—whether your partner, a trusted friend, or a therapist—can often serve to help you purge the toxic residue of such painful encounters.

Talking about Loss

It can also be hard to figure out what to say if you've experienced a miscarriage or an unsuccessful ART attempt. Miscarriage can be excruciating when it comes to the responses of family and friends, because the loss is so misunderstood. A friend who said, "It's for the best," devastated Alana, who miscarried at eight weeks after her first IVF cycle. Even though Alana knew that on some level her friend was trying to comfort her, Alana responded: "Having a miscarriage is not 'for the best'. 'For the best' would be to have a baby!"

If miscarriage is so misunderstood, imagine the reactions to an unsuccessful IVF or other ART intervention. How do you explain that you weren't really pregnant, but you did create an embryo, and you feel the loss just as if you were pregnant? If people question your grief, you might say that you want so much to have a baby and were so close this time, that you felt pregnant, even if not technically so. You can also say, "There's a lot that people don't understand about what it's like to go through these procedures" and leave it at that, or excuse yourself from the conversation by saying that you would rather not talk about it.

People often don't know what to say in these circumstances and may be looking to you for guidance. You may have experienced this awkwardness yourself with others, prior to infertility. Alana admitted that years earlier, her cousin had a miscarriage, and she wasn't sure how to handle it. "I didn't know if I should talk about it or avoid bringing it up," she said. It's even more confusing to know how to talk about IVF.

What we have found is that if you're in the midst of infertility treatment, or have experienced a loss like miscarriage, you aren't looking for advice or helpful hints. Instead, you want others to respect and acknowledge the loss. A simple "I'm sorry," will often suffice. A statement like "It must be so difficult" can be all you need if you are in the midst of IVF. But you might have to teach friends and family that that's what you need. People don't always understand what it means. You may need to explain how real this loss is to you.

Maya, who has a five-year-old daughter, has struggled for two years with secondary infertility. Attempting to comfort her, her mother-in-law said, "You should be thankful that you have one." But this enraged Maya. She replied, "Of course I'm happy I have my daughter; I absolutely adore her. But that doesn't mean I don't want another child. Just because I have one child doesn't mean I'm not upset by my infertility." Her mother-in-law recognized how her comment was off the mark and apologized.

It helps to have ready answers at hand so you are not caught off guard. Of course it is not possible to anticipate every situation that arises, but being prepared can help protect you from falling apart. It won't necessarily take away the sting or the emotional bruises, but having a repertoire of responses helps armor you against feeling helpless and speechless.

Dealing with Your Family

You may feel a special pain when dealing with your parents or in-laws. Remember that part of the wish for a baby may be to provide a grandchild for them, and it can be especially difficult to deal with their disappointment as well as your own.

To Tell or Not

Many parents try to mask their feelings or avoid the topic, but sometimes that backfires. Gwen cringes describing her mother-in-law. "She talks incessantly about her friend's grandchildren," she said. "I can't stand being around her anymore." Although her mother-in-law never questioned her about children, Gwen feels pressured nonetheless by her indirect comments.

Meredith's mother also has not come out and asked Meredith about having kids, but she expresses concern about how hard Meredith is working. "I can read between the lines," Meredith said. "I know she wants me to focus less on my career and more on having a family. She doesn't know that we have been trying, and every time she hints at it, I resist telling her what's going on."

What to tell your family and which family members to confide in depends on all parties involved. There is a delicate balance between their desire to know and your need for privacy. Gwen decided not to disclose anything to her mother-in-law because she knew it would not be held in confidence. She became adept at changing the subject and maintaining a "grin and bear it" attitude. Meredith, tired of feeling angry and defensive with her mother, decided to have a heart-to-heart chat with her. "Once I talked to my mom," Meredith said, "I felt much better. I had been feeling so ashamed, but my mother was very understanding." Meredith made it clear to her mother, however, that she didn't want to discuss the details of the medical procedures, and her mother agreed not to bring up what was going on unless Meredith did.

Discussing your infertility, or not, is yet another situation where the choice is up to you—and there's no right or wrong to what you decide. There may be times when you want to disclose and times when you don't. As discussed in chapter 7, you and your partner need to come to some agreement on how to handle this and stay in tune with each other as time passes.

How much you choose to tell is also up to you and your partner. There is nothing wrong with setting boundaries about what you reveal or what you want to be asked about. In other words, you may decide to tell a family member that you have been trying to get pregnant, but not give medical details. Like Meredith, you can make it clear that you'll talk when you want to, but prefer no prying questions. It depends on the parties involved and your own comfort level. And always know that if a question arises that you aren't willing to discuss, you can simply respond, "That's off limits" or "I don't want to talk about that."

If you do choose to disclose your situation, be aware that at times, the family member you are talking to may not be able to take it all in. This isn't because he or she isn't interested; rather they may be having their own feelings and reactions to your infertility. Leila

noticed that her mother sometimes abruptly changed the topic after
Leila explained the latest procedure she had undergone. Leila eventually realized this wasn't because her mother didn't care, but she
needed some time to understand and let this sink in; she was also
afraid of burdening Leila with her own reactions to such news.

It also may help to imagine how your parents feel learning about
your infertility. Parents sometimes deal with their own emotions by
becoming excessively worried about you. Rather than encouraging
and supporting you as you go through IVF or a corrective surgery,
they may fret about the risks or the stress that treatment creates for
you. This can be difficult to deflect, when you are already anxious.
Remember that your parents feel helpless at not being able to protect their own baby (you!) from pain and suffering.

Asking Your Family for Financial Help

In addition to enlisting your parents' emotional support—if
you choose to—you may consider asking them for financial help,
since the cost of infertility treatment can be exorbitant. In chapter
10, we discuss how money often defines the course of treatment,
but while we're talking about family issues, there can be times
when the money issue comes up—your parents may offer to help
or you might want to ask them for a contribution.

Brandon, a teacher, and his wife Naomi, a nurse, have good
salaries but a small savings account. Their medical insurance covered four IUI procedures, but when none worked, the couple wondered if they should try IVF, which their doctor strongly
recommended. But if they did, how would they pay for it?

"We immediately thought about our parents," Brandon said.
"But how awkward is that? It's not like I'm seventeen asking my fa-

ther for the keys to the car. I'm thirty-five years old, and it doesn't feel right to ask. Especially because I don't know when, if ever, we could pay them back." As discussed in chapter 4, Brandon was feeling the regressive pull of dependency on his parents.

Naomi, who described her family as being very conservative with money, also was in a quandary about approaching them for a loan. "I'm afraid they'll say no. But worse than that, I'm afraid they'll think we are ridiculous for spending so much money on something so risky. The last thing I want from them is a lecture on squandering hard-earned cash. I can hear my father saying, 'Why do you have to spend money on having a baby? Everybody else can do it for free.' "

After much consideration, Brandon and Naomi did decide to go to their families for help. Much to their surprise, their families wanted to help—and offered to give them the money rather than loan it to them.

But parents don't always have the financial resources to help, or if they do, they may not want to lend the money. Asking for financial help may bring up difficult and complicated family dynamics that are unique to each couple and each family. It's important to weigh the cost/benefit ratio of being in debt to your family. Although not a given that there will be negative consequences in asking for financial help, it may affect your relationship with your parents in ways you haven't considered. Will borrowing money give your parents control over you or your treatment decisions? Will they feel entitled to updates on your progress? Will you feel emotionally indebted to them or feel guilty if treatment doesn't work? If you are struggling with keeping your reproductive issues private, you may not want your family involved at all.

Or you may feel awkward about asking for any other help in the future—financial or otherwise.

Adriana's family generously offered to pay for her first IVF treatment. At first, Adriana felt relieved. "Trying to juggle finances became a roadblock to treatment. Gordon and I were stressed about it all the time," Adriana said. "Neither one of us wanted to say no to IVF, but we weren't sure how to cover our costs. So when my parents offered to pay, it seemed like the perfect solution." But when Gordon and Adriana thought it through, they decided not to take the money after all. "It just didn't feel right," she continued. "What if the IVF didn't work? Would they feel obligated to pay for us to try it again? I didn't want to have the feeling that I failed them. I knew I would want to pay them back—not necessarily with money, but with a baby." Adriana and Gordon decided to take a second mortgage on their home instead.

Parental involvement in your treatment can spill over into your relationship with your partner as well. If his parents are willing and able to finance treatment and hers are not, does that make his the better grandparents? What you don't need at this time are disparaging remarks about either side of the family. There's enough tension as it is without feeling as though someone is keeping score, which could also affect your relationships in years to come.

Many couples find it easier to ask several family members for monetary assistance rather than just one. It may feel like less of a burden to spread out the cost. And some couples ask for "matching funds." Knowing that they are contributing half of the cost makes it easier to ask for the other half.

We have found that many families respond positively to requests for help when they have the resources. Your parents also have a reproductive story, which may include becoming grandparents; helping to finance infertility treatment can be a way for them to have their dreams come true as well. But in all cases, such decisions and requests must be carefully discussed, thought out, and planned in a way that respects the feelings, needs, and personalities of everyone involved.

Dealing with the Rest of the World

As we noted earlier, selective perception can make it seem that babies—and the stuff you can buy for them—are everywhere, especially when you are trying to avoid those reminders. When you are feeling particularly vulnerable (after a failed cycle or during that interminable two-week wait or just on a bad day), exposure to children and families can be unbearable.

Going Out and About

Although it is impossible to isolate yourself, when you are feeling particularly down you may want to protect yourself and try to avoid situations where you may be overexposed to children. Again, we're not suggesting that you move to a desert island or isolate yourself to an unhealthy degree, but taking charge of the things you can control (and learning to cope with the things you can't) is perfectly reasonable. You may choose to venture out in the world when it's less likely children will be out and about. Or you may opt to take a different route to work if your usual one takes you past a playground. To avoid seeing so many children while shopping, Denise decided to buy her groceries later at night and go to the mall when it was open late Thursday nights, rather than on the weekends.

Even though you may try your best to avoid infertility-insensitive situations, there are many times—as when Monique went to the cooking class or Kathleen went to the new doctor—when you simply can't. As you know, reminders of infertility are everywhere you turn. On her way to purchase a new toaster oven, Raquel passed a maternity clothing store. "My heart sank as I glanced at the window display. I didn't want to break down right then and there, but I could feel myself welling up."

What can you do in a situation like this? Again, recognize that your feelings are normal. So often, it's when you least expect it that you get jolted by the family-centric world we live in. When this happens, it's only natural that you will feel awful, as Raquel did. You can choose to go home if possible, put on a stiff upper lip and go on with your business, use self-talk to boost yourself, or sometimes, as Raquel did that day, let yourself have a good cry. "Although I didn't want to cry in public," Raquel said, "I felt so much better after I did."

Remember that *Free to be You and Me* song lyric, "It's all right to cry"? Unfortunately too many of us forget that and view crying as a sign of weakness. We tend to be embarrassed by tears; the crier feels more vulnerable, and those around her feel it's their job to stop the tears. But crying is necessary—it is a healthy release of tension, anger, and frustration, even if tears well up at inopportune moments. It's essential to shed tears to grieve all the losses you have endured because of infertility.

Socializing

Social situations also can inundate you with family and kid stuff. Social gatherings of friends or family—even if they are for adults only—often revolve around children. Someone talks about a baby-sitter who was late, or the new school their child has started, or how their little one just learned to walk. As we discussed in chapter 5, children are extensions of a parent's self; it's no wonder that parents boast about their kids.

But these situations make infertile couples feel bad and out of place. What might have been fun in the past now may feel like a dreaded obligation. As Rhoda described: "At one moment I may really feel like going to a party, while the next I want to shutter all the windows and never go out again. It's been a long three years." This normal and to-be-expected ambivalence about social events hits every infertile person at some time or another. And it's likely to be stronger when you've had bad news or are feeling low, because you are more sensitive and fragile at those moments.

In handling social obligations, we need to emphasize once again that there is no right or wrong way to approach social functions; it's your choice whether to attend or not. There may be events that ordinarily you would never miss—a friend's baby shower or your family's Thanksgiving feast—but they may be too painful to go to in your present circumstances. Be careful not to get caught up in the "shoulds." Part of Rhoda's ambivalence is tied up with her feeling she's supposed to socialize.

It is perfectly okay not to attend everything you are invited to—especially baby showers, children's birthday parties, or holiday events focused on family and children. You can say, "I'm sorry, we'd love to, but we've already made other plans." If you do say yes, but at the last minute change your mind, give yourself permission to cancel. You need to take care of yourself, even if you disappoint a friend or relative.

As we discussed previously, the holidays can be a particularly stressful time, with so much emphasis and attention placed on family. You may want to consider making alternate plans to reduce emotional stress. Many of our clients opt to go on vacation during the holidays. Others decide to have a quiet dinner at home and celebrate privately.

It's not always easy to change family traditions. Your family may not understand why you don't want to be with them, or may take your not attending personally. You worry or feel guilty that you will hurt their feelings. As much as we wish it otherwise, sometimes that is unavoidable. Be prepared to field their reactions, but realize you cannot always make it better for them. You need to take care of yourself during this crisis, and at some point, accept that your family members will have to handle their own feelings and they will eventually get over it.

If you have to go to an event, how should you handle it? There may be times when your partner wants to socialize, but you don't, or vice versa. Try to find a balance and a compromise so both your needs can be met. You can decide to go separately, or you can choose to arrive late and/or leave early to limit the trauma you may feel. Also, we recommend that you and your partner have a pre-arranged set of cues or signals to let each other know if one of you begins to feel upset or overwhelmed while you are out.

"We were at my cousin's house for Easter," said Roger, "and I saw Mandy cornered by my eighty-five-year-old Aunt Betty, who is well-meaning but can talk your ear off. Poor Mandy was trying to be nice to my aunt, but I could tell by her body language that Mandy needed to get away." So he stepped in and rescued her from his aunt.

If you're stuck in an awkward conversation, excuse yourself to retreat to the rest room or leave the party. "I'm not feeling well" is an easy way out. And if you and your partner can keep an eye out for each other, that can be a lifesaver.

Dealing with Friends

"My best friend Linda just announced she's pregnant," Chelsea, who has had two chemical pregnancies, said. "That's the third one of my friends to get pregnant this year. They are all so happy that it makes me feel my own sadness more deeply. To make things worse, I feel like such a terrible friend—why can't I even be happy for Linda?"

As you know all too well, it's easy to feel like the odd woman out and become isolated from your closest friends. And it's difficult to want to feel happy for them but realize that you just don't—that instead you feel remarkably sorry for yourself. You want to do the right thing with your friend and congratulate her, yet how do you do the right thing for yourself?

With close friends, you may want to open up and share what you're going through, as you might with a trusted family member. It can be more comforting than you expect, in part because you may learn that others in your circle have shared your experience, but never talked about it.

Sometimes, though, you may find that talking about what you are going through with a friend doesn't work. Your friend may not understand or may not be able to handle your pain. It can feel like a betrayal when you confide in someone, only to have your friend change the subject, or worse, talk about someone else who just got pregnant.

It can feel awkward to confront your friend and share that you are angry or hurt by their response. But it might be better to get your hurt feelings out in the open than let them build up inside and feed a growing resentment that could doom the friendship. It can also be a way of educating your friend—most people, when made aware of their painful actions, will learn from their mistakes.

How the conflict resolves may depend on how open and close the friendship has been. Is it okay to let your friend know how you're feeling? You bet. But if you find that they are not able to respond positively, you may need to limit the relationship until you feel better. Right now, it is more important to take care of yourself, even to the point of temporarily suspending a relationship, than it is to nurture a friendship that brings you mostly pain. It's the sad truth that some friendships will dissolve over infertility, although many can be resumed at a later date. While this is painful, please don't berate yourself if you find yourself needing time and space away from a friend who hurts you more than helps.

How Do I Handle this at Work?

"I think there is a population explosion going on in our company," said Marion, a personnel director of a large corporation. She and her husband, Walt, have been trying for two years. "In this past year alone, there have been eight births, and three more women are pregnant. Last week there was an office baby shower, which was hard enough to sit through, when one of the guys jokingly asked me when it was going to be my turn. I smiled, said, 'It'll be a while' and tried to shrug it off as another stupid thing that another stupid person said—but inside I was ready to spit daggers."

How do you handle these interactions at work? These are tough situations—you see these people every day and may spend more time with them than good friends, yet you may not want everyone in your workplace to know you're struggling with infertility. "People talk," Marion said. "I know because I hear it all the time. The last thing I need is for people gossiping about me or pitying me. This is private and it needs to stay that way, but it's not easy." The cheerful mask Marion wears at work feels ready to crack, especially at vulnerable moments.

At times like these, Marion needs to remember that her infertility is not who she is as a person. Being cared about is not the same as being pitied, or gossiped about. She needs to be prepared to tell people that she would rather not talk about it, but recognize that she cannot control how others think and feel about her. Venting to someone outside of work can provide a much-needed release.

It's also incredibly upsetting if you trust and confide in someone, only to hear about it later from someone else. This can happen at work or with friends or family. Sylvia told a work colleague, in confidence, why she needed time off work; it felt better to her than hiding what was going on. At lunch a few days later, however, she was shocked when a different co-worker started talking about an infertile friend who got pregnant when she went on vacation. "It was a double whammy," Sylvia raged. "Not only was her advice ridiculous, but I knew the only way she could have known about my situation was by talking to my colleague. It was such a betrayal—I couldn't believe it."

The feelings that Marion and Sylvia bring to light are not isolated cases. Unfortunately, they happen all the time—in the workplace and outside of it. Like Marion and Sylvia, you may find it helpful to discuss your anger and hurt with someone you can trust—be it a spouse, a friend, a support group, or a therapist. Using your infertility diary at these times is also an excellent way to release your feelings.

When Dealing with the World Becomes Overwhelming

While we hope that the suggestions in this chapter help you cope with everyday situations, we also encourage you to look elsewhere for help when you feel isolated and confused by your feelings. Support groups, Web sites, and therapists can all help during these trying times.

Warning Signs You Can't Ignore

Before we proceed, a word of caution: during infertility trauma, sometimes the stress you're experiencing can turn into clinical depression, in which case it is important that you seek professional help. Here are warning signs that you should get help from a mental health professional:

- crying all the time (not just sometimes)
- being unable to get out of bed (more than occasionally)
- feeling unable to concentrate (not just now and then)
- having suicidal ideas (even if no plan)

Your primary-care physician, your gynecologist, and your infertility specialists are all good referral sources.

Often, a course of antidepressant medication can help. Many women resist taking any medication because they worry about the potential effects on the baby and research on this issue is still ongoing. But depression, which can lead to not eating or sleeping properly, may pose substantial risks during pregnancy. In some cases, the risk of *not* taking antidepressants may outweigh the risks of taking them. It's essential to consult with a psychiatrist or other physician who can make the best recommendations for your particular situation.

Support Groups

Fortunately, there are many support groups specifically for infertile couples, and in the appendix we've compiled a list of organizations that sponsor groups. Support groups have different focuses and topics—some are women only, others are for couples, or those experiencing secondary infertility. You will be able to meet others who are in similar situations to receive comfort and support. If you are not comfortable in a group situation, there are also numerous Internet bulletin boards and Web sites where you can anonymously discuss your situation.

Support groups and Web sites provide reassurance and acknowledgment that you are not alone. They offer a venue for airing your feelings; it is comforting to know that other people will understand your experience because they are experiencing it too. Having a sense of belonging, which infertile couples struggle with so much, is encouraging, even if this is not the "club" you had hoped or expected to join.

When choosing a support group, please consider whether or not the group is led by a professional moderator. A professional can help group members understand the psychological complexity of their experiences and provide referrals if further help is needed. As we discuss below, they can also help group members keep a handle on the feelings that can occur when someone in the group becomes pregnant or has a procedure fail.

While support groups can be highly beneficial, they do have some pitfalls. It's wonderful to have a group to commiserate with, but what happens when someone in the group gets pregnant? Before, everyone was on the same side of the fence, but when someone gets pregnant that group member moves to the other side. Once again, there is a sense of not belonging anymore. Even the couple who has become pregnant may feel uneasy and not know how to manage their relationships within the group. This can make the group feel strained and awkward. Here a professional moderator can help—what works well is if the group can openly discuss these issues. Then, if and when the situation occurs, everyone is prepared to deal with it.

Likewise, the Internet has its own drawbacks. It can be a valuable resource, but it is easy to be overwhelmed by the vast amount of information. While we don't discourage our clients from using the Internet, we do caution them to pace themselves and not to take everything they read at face value. On bulletin boards, for example, people share experiences and advice, but misinformation also abounds. It's fine to ask your e-friends questions, but always confirm what you learn with your physician. Sometimes, it helps to set a time limit for your Web surfing. Information can help to manage anxiety, but becoming obsessed with Web searches and bulletin boards can be counterproductive.

Therapy

Sometimes couples need more individual support than talking with family, friends, or fellow group members. It can be enormously valuable for infertile individuals and couples to seek professional help through this rough period. It's not uncommon for people to worry that seeking therapy means that something more is wrong with them, at a time when their self-esteem is already under assault from infertility. But remember that infertility is a unique trauma that goes outside the range of what we expect in life. Not only can therapy ease your own burden, but it can have an effect on your partner as well. Even if men don't want to see a therapist (unfortunately, not an atypical reaction) they can benefit from what their wives learn. It can take the strain out of those times in your marriage when you really need someone to talk to and your partner is not, or cannot be, available.

Candace felt she was unraveling at the seams after her first IVF was unsuccessful. "The doctor tried to reassure me that many IVFs fail on the first try. She said, 'Now we know how your body reacts to the medications; trial number two will be that much better.' " Candace understood this rationally, but emotionally she still needed to vent. "It's not just this IVF, but all the other stuff we have gone through over the past four years—and also what we are facing next. I know I won't be judged in therapy. I can get it all off my chest—whatever it is—and I'm not going to burden anyone else with this."

People feel better after they are able to put into words what has been stirring inside of them. It's as if you have an in-box full of work that keeps staring you in the face and driving you crazy. Giving voice to your feelings is like getting some of that work done. Talking about it takes the contents of the "to be done" file (what has been banging around inside of you and causing so much grief) and puts it all in the "finished" file (literally getting it out of you).

Many times, the work is not so much completed as it is a work in progress, but it is the process of getting it out from inside of you that relieves so much of the burden.

Therapy is unique in that it establishes a confidential and non-judgmental environment—it is a safe space for you to explore your feelings about your infertility trauma. Being able to vent and blow off steam to someone who is supportive and caring is similar to having a good cry. And you may feel safer shedding tears or expressing anger to someone trained to handle those feelings, someone who can normalize your experience and help you understand it.

As therapists and as therapy patients ourselves, we encourage you to develop as deep an understanding of the psychological effects of infertility as possible. The more you know and understand about yourself and the effects of infertility, the better you will feel. This goes for your partner as well. The more the two of you can identify the sources of your feelings, appreciate your individual ways of coping and grieving, and your unique reproductive stories, the more you can give each other support without feeling misunderstood.

If you decide to pursue therapy, choose a therapist who is knowledgeable about the issues related to infertility. Look for a therapist who listens well and does not have preconceived opinions on how your reproductive story should unfold. Psychiatrists, psychologists, social workers, and other licensed professionals can offer individual and marital psychotherapy. Specific credentials matter less than finding a well-trained therapist experienced in the sensitive issues regarding reproductive trauma and loss. Shop around if you need to, but don't just pick a name from the phone book; ask your doctors, your friends who are also going through this, and your support group leader for referrals. The right therapist can provide a safe haven, a place where you can feel accepted and understood, and where you can put the pieces of your personal puzzle back together again.

You Are Coping, Even Though it May Not Feel Like it

There is no way around the fact that infertility is a life-altering event. The world no longer feels like such a welcoming place, and you may not feel very safe navigating it every day. Infertility changes how you think about yourself and how you deal with others. How you interact with your family, friends and co-workers, with the world in general, is not the same as it once was. Learning how to cope in an environment that is so family-focused is a challenge, to say the least.

As you struggle to find your footing, please keep in mind that it's all right to laugh, or cry, or get angry; it's all right to feel all the crazy things you're feeling. Feeling one way in the morning and another in the evening is not only okay, it's to be expected. It's all right to hide when you need to, just as it's all right to reach out to others. You are not alone in this—although it often feels as if you are.

While wanting a family and going to enormous lengths to achieve this goal is the center of your life right now, remember that it is only one part of who you are. As we mentioned before, infertility may be a gigantic piece of the puzzle of who you are, but it is still only one piece. That's why we encourage self-talk when you feel down—it's a tool to keep infertility separate from the rest of who you are. Reminding yourself of your strengths when you feel so vulnerable can be hard. But it can also boost your self-esteem, giving you the energy you need to get through any number of tough situations.

And never forget the power of your sense of humor. Though you may not feel like laughing now, much of this process—if you can step far away enough from it—can be strangely funny. Even through your tears, try to keep in perspective the absurdity of it all. After Raquel cried in front of the maternity store, she chuckled about it later when she was home. "Of all the different routes I could have taken to get to the appliance store," she said, "I had to pick the one that would land me right in the middle of it all. Geez, talk about a sense of direction!" Letting yourself laugh about all this is as important as letting yourself cry.

PART IV

Rewriting Your Reproductive Story

Ten

Knowing When to Stop Trying

One of the most profound decisions an infertile couple must make—as important as the decision to try to conceive in the first place—is the decision to stop trying. You may feel as if you'll never know when to stop. You may not even be ready to consider this yet. Or perhaps the question of when to stop is initially popping up in your mind.

This decision isn't always crystal clear; you can feel much uncertainty and confusion at what your next move should be. At one moment, you may be ready to stop, the next you're ready to try again. And it's not always clear what stopping means. For some, stopping means limiting infertility treatment. For others, it means no longer actively pursuing treatment for a biological child. So are you stopping your effort to conceive naturally? Are you stopping taking medications such as Clomid? Are you ceasing the IUIs? Or are you stopping IVF? When do you stop trying?

Wherever you are in your journey, we encourage you to consider carefully how you feel about going on at every stage of the process. Too often, in a haze of stress and anxiety, you move on blindly, without considering the ramifications of your next move. Yet ART, as remarkable as it is, carries with it a number of moral and spiritual dilemmas, to say nothing of the financial cost that you must factor into your decision about whether or not to continue. Of course, the decision about whether or not to stop also depends on what your doctor says; you'll need to find out all you can about treatment options and what's right for you medically. These issues can complicate the decision process, so it's important that you confront and discuss these issues head on.

In this chapter, we explore the emotional issues and dilemmas you may face as you pursue infertility treatment and try to decide which interventions are right for you. We also discuss how to determine when "enough is enough" psychologically and what happens when you finally make the decision to stop trying.

It can be agonizingly difficult to face not having a biological child. And when you do make that decision, there are still more decisions to be made. In chapter 11, we explore how couples come to terms with rewriting their reproductive stories, incorporating the story lines of becoming a parent through alternate means—such as using donor eggs or sperm, a surrogate, or pursuing adoption—or deciding to be childfree.

You Made a Choice to Start, You Make a Choice to Stop

It's often hard to figure out when to stop treatment because the infertility treatment process becomes all-consuming. Not only are you and your partner on an emotional and medical roller coaster, the process of infertility treatment can make you feel stuck on a treadmill with no off-switch. You keep trudging ahead as the myriad treatment options feed the hope that "if we try just one more time, that will be the one that works."

Your longing for a baby can pull you deeper into infertility treatment than you would ever have imagined when you first started. "I was horrified when my doctor suggested that I take a little Clomid to help me ovulate," said Sally. "I was one of those people who hated taking medicine. Now, here I am three years, six IUIs, and two IVFs later, still not pregnant. I can't quite believe this. But I want a baby so much, how can I say no when there is a chance it will work?"

So many of our clients are exhausted by their treatment, and like Sally, feel conflicted about their decisions but compelled to go on. Are you feeling this way too? You keep making treatment decisions as you try and try again to have a baby; various doors either open or close as you and your doctor learn more about your body and how it responds to treatment. And all of this happens with the added pressure of time passing hanging over your head.

Assuming there's no medical contraindication, it's okay to take short breaks off the treatment treadmill. Taking off a month or two—or even six—can clear your head and refuel you, particularly when you are feeling bewildered and unsure of what to do next. Slow down to give yourself a chance to listen to your body, mind, and spirit.

By releasing the valve on the pressure cooker of treatment, you consider your options more clearly. Of course your feelings and plans may seesaw from one day to the next, but with a break you have the time and space to think about what next steps seem best for you, or establish a time frame for how long you will pursue a particular treatment.

Remember, just as you made a choice to start infertility treatments, you can make the choice to continue treatments or to stop them.

Your Reproductive Story

Whether the decision to stop trying seems clear-cut or not, many important feelings arise at this juncture of the reproductive story. It's critical to explore and acknowledge how your reproductive story is changing—and how you feel about those changes.

Part of the challenge in deciding which treatments you want to pursue, and how many times, is that the path to parenthood has many components. The aspects of parenthood that are most important to you play a role in determining the interest or comfort level you have with any type of treatment.

- Is the act of conception the most important part, meaning that you are only comfortable becoming a parent if you can conceive "the old-fashioned way"?
- Is having a biological child the most important? If so, then you might be willing to relinquish your wish to conceive "naturally" and use IUIs or IVF, if it would mean that the baby carried your and your partner's genetic selves.
- Or is having the experience of pregnancy the most essential piece of your story, even if the child is not genetically yours and your partner's? If that is the case, then donor technology of sperm, egg, or both might be options that you would consider.
- If having a biological child is more important than pregnancy and birth then you might consider using a surrogate

to carry your embryos, or your husband's sperm and a donor egg.

- Or if you realize that the most important part is to have a baby to parent, regardless of its biological roots, then adoption might be the answer.

As you consider these questions, figure out what feels right for you—again, there are no right or wrong answers. Some couples taper off treatment or let their various options overlap, such as beginning the adoption process while continuing with another IVF or IUI. This may help you from feeling too invested in any one route, and less devastated by the setbacks, since you know what your next step will be.

The Finances of Infertility

Infertility is financially as well as physically draining. As you well know, the cost of infertility treatment can be exorbitant. Insurance coverage varies: some health insurers cover only the tests for diagnosis, some cover certain aspects of treatment but not others, while other plans may set a dollar limit on payments for infertility treatment. Figuring out the finances of ART is another confusing and overwhelming ordeal for infertile couples.

Even in the rare instance when insurance covers IVF cycles, most couples have to pay for some part, if not all, of their treatment expenses, such as co-pays or medications. You may be in the position to pay for these procedures yourself, but many couples need to borrow money or go into debt. Financial considerations often define the course of treatment.

Balancing your longing for a baby with the other economic de-

mands of life is tricky business. Couples often make great sacrifices in order to pay for treatment—do you put off buying a new
car? Not go on vacation? A choice in the service of one need or life
milestone may undermine another. Lillian and Kevin, after a year
of unsuccessful interventions to clear her blocked tubes, must now
decide whether to spend their savings on a house down payment or
an IVF cycle. "We thought it would be great to live near Lillian's
sister and husband," Kevin said. "They've got a six-month-old; we
thought we'd have one by now too. We thought we'd baby-sit for
each other and raise our families together." They ultimately chose
to defer on their dream of a house, and spend part of their down
payment on their IVF.

As a couple, you'll grapple with tough issues figuring out how to
finance your treatments. It's critical that you and your partner be
honest about what resources you have, what options are available,
where you might be able to sacrifice. Maybe, as we discussed in
chapter 9, you'll decide to approach your families for help.

Is this Investment Worth it?

It's also important to recognize that not only are large sums involved, the outcome of this expense is by no means guaranteed.
People vary in their response to financial risk, and if you are
spending a nest egg or taking out a second mortgage, you may feel
extremely anxious. If your partner experiences financial risk differently, it can fuel a struggle over whose values should be honored.

Lance, who grew up in a home where money was very tight,
worries about "running out of cash." His wife, Jenny, thinks that
even if money is tight now, she and Lance can make more later. In
the course of arguing, they realized that their disagreement

stemmed from their conflicting attitudes toward money, not their actual financial resources. By talking this through, they agreed to spend a certain amount on treatment, and then continue their discussion when they reached that cap. Lance felt better with a limit established; Jenny felt the amount reflected what they could afford to spend now.

How Can You Place a Price Tag on a Baby?

Yet another tricky feeling can creep into your discussions about treatment costs. Some people struggle because they worry that they are "buying a baby," when they must pay ten or twenty thousand dollars (or more) for an IVF cycle.

Jane and Tim, who have been undergoing treatments for four years, still argue about the costs. "We want a baby—there's no doubt about that, but it is killing us financially. How do you put a price tag on making a family? How much is 'too much' to spend? Tim wants to stop, but I feel like if we don't keep trying, we'll feel like we didn't do everything we could."

Figuring Out What to Spend

We advise our clients to consider the expense in the context of the bigger picture of their life. Did you take out a college loan that you repaid over many years? Perhaps if you think of infertility treatment as an investment in your future, much like a college education, it might be easier to accept. Even education loans can take years to pay back. "But it might not work!" you exclaim. That's true, and in that regard, infertility is even more like an investment, in that it carries some degree of financial risk. But so does a college education. What if you go to college and major in business and then decide you want to be a teacher instead and have to go back to school? Does that make your degree a waste? Of course not. Infertility treatment is not guaranteed, but it buys you an opportunity that you may not have otherwise.

Knowing when to stop spending is a highly personal decision, which depends on your resources and your ability as a couple to tolerate the anxiety that accompanies financial risk. This is an investment gamble—you may be spending money and still not have a baby to show for it. But it is an opportunity.

Finally, it's okay to feel resentful that you have to pay so much for what others do for free. It can be hard to accept that this all costs so much—that doctors and clinics are making money from all these invasive tests and procedures. You may find yourself feeling ambivalent about the business aspects of your doctor's practice. This is understandable. What is a professional business for them feels like the key to your future. But try to stay focused on the task at hand and the services your doctor provides. Most doctors work to create soothing, comfortable environments for their patients, with the best possible equipment and services.

It is also the case, however, that being charged for every single step in the process—whether it works or not—is very stressful. There's no harm in asking for a discount if you've gone back to a doctor or clinic for repeated cycles. If your insurance doesn't cover medications, sometimes clinics have extra medications on hand or programs where other patients donate unused meds. It's worth asking. Some people feel embarrassed or needy by asking for a break; it's yet another affront to their self-esteem. But doctors are aware of the financial strain these procedures can cause and may be willing to discuss their fees with you.

Spiritual Considerations

Feeling Guilty

"I never considered myself to be that religious," noted Marilyn. "But thinking about using ART, I am having second thoughts. Maybe I'm not supposed to have a child. Maybe God has a plan for me and I just don't know what it is."

Marilyn had never believed in fate as the driving force of her life, but infertility has made her question basic beliefs. "My mother says that only God can make a baby and if it isn't happening, it's because I haven't been strong enough in my faith." At first, Marilyn was furious with her mother for making her feel guilty, but now she's not so sure. "I don't know what I believe anymore."

Many people face tough religious and spiritual questions as they consider ART. And the despair and confusion you feel about your infertility can also spur mixed feelings about your faith.

Some people, like Marilyn, worry that they are "playing God" when they pursue infertility treatment. These spiritual dilemmas about ART may not coincide with the other ways you view medicine or religion. You may feel no compunction about using other medical technology, but draw the line when it comes to reproductive technology. A person who believes that medical knowledge was provided or inspired by God may become anxious when considering infertility treatment. Why should reproductive technology be any different from other medical technology? The anxiety and fear of judgment may reflect one's own sense of guilt and shame about being infertile. People define themselves by their reproductive capacities in ways that they simply do not if they have a problem with some other body part. The anxiety evoked regarding religion may also speak, to some extent, to the deep roots of their reproductive story, with its beginnings in early childhood. People may bring an almost childlike fear to their images and perceptions of God and church when it comes to reproductive issues. They worry that they will be judged harshly, even when their adult selves know better. It's as if their infertility means that they are fundamentally bad or lacking, and that the church will view them that way as well.

When you are struggling with the moral or religious aspects of infertility, you may also tend to rewrite history. You only remember what you've done wrong in the eyes of your religion; you recall "bad" past deeds or thoughts or past sexual behavior. Infertility becomes a self-indictment, a punishment for the errors you feel you have made in the past—even if the decisions were thoughtful and resolved at the time. The self-judgment and spiritual issues can become interwoven with your own anxieties; your fear of reprisals from religious leaders or the congregation may reflect your own judgment of yourself. In your mind, infertility turns into a punishment from God, rather than a medical crisis.

Feeling Abandoned or Angry at God

Some people may feel angry with or abandoned by God—and then feel guilty about their doubts. Brad, a highly religious man who volunteers at his church, had an alcoholic father who vanished when Brad was eleven years old. "I've tried to be a good person," Brad said. "I grew up fast. I've worked since I was fourteen trying to help my mother make ends meet. I swore I would never let something like that happen when I became a dad." Brad did things "right" and yet still has no kids of his own. "Yes, I'm angry with God," he continued. "How could a loser like my father get to be a father, and I can't? Where's the justice in that?" Abandoned by his father at a young age, now Brad feels abandoned by God.

It is important to remember that your psychological and spiritual selves are closely bound, and that it is natural to question, to grieve, and to want to blame something outside yourself for your misfortune. Tracy wondered, "Why me? Why wasn't God helping me out in all of this?" Tracy came to realize that, in her depression over her seven years of infertility, she had stopped seeing the world as a good and just place. "I forgot about all the blessings that I do have. God hasn't pushed me away—I have retreated." Comforted by her recognition that her relationship with God was, like so much else, a highly personal, internal experience, Tracy felt less alone.

Those who don't consider themselves religious may also question their belief system. When Edie felt desperate about having a baby, she was surprised to find herself praying. "I'm not exactly sure I was praying to God, but I closed my eyes and whispered, 'Please, please, let this work.' It was so automatic." For Edie, praying expressed her hope that someone or something outside of herself could help her.

Is Yours a Loving God?

In working with people on these spiritual issues, we encourage them to think about their particular God—and to clarify for themselves whether they see God as loving or judgmental. We ask them to consider why a loving God would punish them for wanting to have a baby. If they feel that God forgives them for whatever sin they feel they committed in the past, why can they not forgive themselves?

We also encourage people to try to separate their personal views of God from formal religious doctrine when they are considering these issues. This can help them clarify if their anxiety reflects their true spiritual beliefs or if it has more to do with their fears of being judged by their social community, family members, or by themselves.

We also encourage you to speak with your spiritual leader about your concerns. Often you will receive more support than you expected.

Am I Selfish for Using ART?

"There is something about creating a baby with assistance that doesn't seem right to me," Melanie said, who has been trying for three years. "I desperately want to be pregnant and give birth, but maybe I should adopt a child who has no other opportunities. It seems selfish not to adopt. Am I wrong for wanting my own?"

You too may be struggling with feeling selfish about using ART. A little voice inside your head nags: *Why aren't you adopting instead? There are lots of babies who need homes.* And you may feel pressure from family members and friends who suggest that you "just adopt."

But self-criticism and guilt about wishing to be pregnant—like for Melanie—makes it all the more difficult for you to comfortably move forward with medical treatment—or decide to stop. We talk to many couples who feel that they "should" do something and yet struggle with the feeling that they don't want to. These feelings about using ART may reflect deeper narcissistic wounds and shame about being infertile. It's helpful to separate feelings about yourself from the specifics of your decision, so that you do not unduly punish or deprive yourself of what you truly want.

At any stage of this process, it's crucial that your decisions be made without remorse or guilt attached. If you want to keep on with treatment, by all means do. Adoption is a wonderful choice, but to adopt and deny yourself medical treatment out of guilt is not constructive for yourself or the baby you are adopting. If and when you choose to adopt, do so because you want to, not because you think you should.

Impossible Decisions

As you move through the treatment process, you also need to acknowledge the risks and concerns raised by ART—the impossible decisions you may have to face if you get pregnant. While every pregnancy is inherently risky, using ART may present you with a higher instance of complicated circumstances. Women over the age of thirty-five are at a greater risk of miscarriage and genetic anomalies. ART also increases the likelihood of multiple births, which can increase the risk to both mother and babies.

It's important to recognize that this medical technology, which may give us our only opportunity to have a baby, also can present us with difficult and agonizing choices. Consider that diagnostic tests such as ultrasound and amniocentesis provide you with information that in the past wouldn't have been available.

Of course, no one knows what decisions you'll have to make if you do become pregnant. But it is important to recognize the potential risks and decisions involved. What might you do if amniocentesis results come back badly? What might you do if you find yourself pregnant with three or more embryos? How you might handle these difficult and complicated decisions may inform your treatment decisions.

Each individual and couple will have to decide what is right for them. But it's important to face these questions as you consider how far to go with treatment. It's best to gather information, talk to your doctors, consult with genetic counselors, and search within yourself to prepare for different scenarios. It is not a matter of expecting the worst, but of being realistic and prepared for the risks involved with ART.

What Makes it So Hard to Stop

Like a gambler hoping for a win, infertile couples find themselves enticed by the lure of "one more time." What if the next try, that new procedure, this different clinic really will be the ticket to a successful outcome? It's so hard to turn your back on that possibility, especially when you hear about other people's successful attempts.

Sara heard about a new doctor through her support group. Only thirty-four, she has been told by two different doctors after two IVFs that she's an under-responder and simply does not produce enough eggs. Still reluctant to accept her diagnosis, she can't help but be excited about a new doctor. "Everyone was raving about him and I thought, 'I've got to go see him too.' I know my husband won't be thrilled. He's had it! He's been hinting around about adoption—he told me last night about a work friend who adopted—but what if this doctor really can help us? I don't think I could stand it if we close the door right now."

With a carrot dangling in front of you, enticing you to try yet another doctor and yet another procedure, it is no wonder stop-ping can be hard to do. Sara is not alone in not wanting to leave any stone unturned. Combine that with a natural instinct to achieve what we have set out to do, and we have a formula that keeps us going for a very long time.

Knowing When Enough Is Enough

Some couples set limits right from the start; they know which treatments they are willing to undergo and which they are not. Or they know their insurance covers a certain number of procedures so that's their limit. When they have tried all the interventions they set out to do, they know it's the right time to stop.

Most others don't know—or find their "limits" changing as they go through the treatment process. For many couples, the decision to stop is driven by finances. Few of us have unlimited resources to dedicate to infertility treatment. And if you are considering other options—like adoption, surrogacy, or donor technology—those re-quire a significant financial investment as well.

Other couples stop actively trying for a biological child when their emotional resources run dry. As you well know, it is exhaust-ing to go through one loss after another. The wear and tear on your soul as well as your body is tremendous. And if you are thinking about other avenues to parenthood, it is important to stop when you still have some emotional energy to devote to your next steps.

Trisha knew exactly when her emotional coffers were empty. "I saw a robin build her nest last spring, watched her sit on the nest, and couldn't wait to see the baby birds. But one day the robin was gone. When I went outside to look, I found shells broken on the ground. I sobbed and sobbed. I knew right then that I was at my emotional tipping point. I couldn't go on with any more treatment; it was time to move on."

The physical drain is another factor to consider. The hormones and other medications you take place great strain on your body. You feel bloated, out of sorts, not yourself. While many of the surgical procedures are "routine," they all have their risks, and those requiring anesthesia have even more. As Trisha added: "If I never have to go into a hospital again, it will be too soon!"

Even if you've known for sure that you always were going to stop after two IVF cycles, the decision to stop can be an emotional and painful one. Not only are you rewriting your reproductive story—deciding not to try any longer for your own biological child—you are likely also feeling vulnerable, worn out, and still a bit stressed and depressed. No wonder that making another major life change—to stop trying—is difficult.

Waving the White Flag

Wrestling with the decision to stop treatment may bring up feelings of defeat. After fighting a valiant battle, it is time to retreat, but you may have an uncomfortable feeling that you are quitting. All of us are too familiar with the cliché, "If at first you don't succeed, try, try again." It's so deeply ingrained that letting go of this "project" may give rise to a sense of failure.

Sometimes people choose to continue trying to avoid feeling sadness or grief. It may be easier to hold onto the identity of "infertility patient" than to feel that you have reached the end of the road.

As your treatment has progressed, you have already come to

terms with being in a place you never thought you'd be in. With each option you gain something—new hope, another chance—but you also lose something: the lost opportunity from the procedure that didn't work. In a weird way, you move farther from your goal of parenthood even as you move forward to the next technique.

The decision to stop treatment encompasses yet another level of loss that couples must mourn. For some, it is only now, when you step off the treadmill for good, that you can finally begin your grieving process. In its own way, being in the coping mode for so long may have protected you from the full effects of this trauma; there was no time before to grieve. So be prepared for a potentially big crash when you decide to stop.

Paul and Donna knew from the get-go that they didn't want to do IVF; they felt it was too risky and expensive. But when they reached their self-imposed stopping point, Paul was besieged with questions regarding what to do next. The only son of an only son, he felt responsible to carry on his genetic line. Donna, while sad about not experiencing a pregnancy and not having a biological child, was ready to proceed with adoption.

"I'm having a hard time understanding how Donna can be so happy about this," Paul said. "She has already started writing a letter to introduce us to prospective birth mothers. I know we agreed that we wouldn't do IVF, but this is happening too fast."

Like many infertility patients, Paul's drive to continue treatment was his way to circumvent the crash; he wasn't yet ready to give up his dream of having a biological child and wanted to avoid the loss he would inevitably face. Yet he felt relieved when he realized he was experiencing a normal phase of grief—the denial phase. "I finally understand that my push to continue medical interventions was an evasive maneuver. It was my way of avoiding the obvious need to say good-bye to my dreams."

Coming to this realization, Paul was able to grieve his hopes for a biological child. And as he did so, he shifted the story line of his reproductive story and joined his wife on the path to adoption. His decision now felt proactive and positive rather than a defeat.

Giving Yourself Permission to Stop

It's okay to stop treatment. But it's important to realize that some outside pressures may make you feel you "should" go on. We've noticed many times that a couple deciding whether or not to stop treatment will start talking about what their friends are doing, how that infertile couple is trying their sixth IVF cycle or is trying yet another new treatment protocol.

It's easy to compare yourself to others and feel yourself coming up short—as if this were a true test of your strength and stamina. You may even feel angry or jealous of friends if they have the means (emotional or financial) to continue treatment when you're not sure you can go on. Being aware of these unconscious comparisons can help you avoid a "keeping up with the Joneses" attitude.

What's right for one couple is not necessarily right for another. It's natural when you hear about what someone else is doing—what new technique they have tried—to think that you should try it too, but question that automatic reaction. "Well, if they can hang in there, then we should be able to"—that's a burden that can interfere with your personal decision-making. When talking to other couples, also keep in mind that your decision to stop might be threatening to those in the same boat as you.

The decision to stop is yours alone and is particular to your diagnosis, experience, and circumstances. When you are feeling uncertain about how to proceed, it may help to consult with your doctor, to review the medical options and recommendations once again. If you are having difficulty deciding what to do, by all means seek a second or third opinion if that will help. At the same time, know that the decision to stop treatment is not one that a doctor can always make for you. He or she may recommend another procedure, and even encourage you to continue, but ultimately, you must decide what is best for you.

Just because you can do something does not mean that you should do it. It is important to give yourself permission to stop, just as you initially gave yourself permission to seek treatment.

Who Am I Now? Who Will I Be?

Part of the challenge of making treatment decisions is that with each step we change the way we think about ourselves. Remember that initial shift from healthy and normal to "infertility patient"? So what happens when you are no longer an infertility patient? Even though you may have disliked aspects of your treatment, the process did provide structure and progress that could be comforting, or that at least became familiar.

After spending so much time engrossed in your treatment and diagnosis, your identity is being jolted again. This shift—from being on the ride to getting off—can feel like a relief, but can also feel confusing. Once again, you must figure out who you are, what you want, and where you fit in.

"When I finally got off that interminable infertility treadmill,"

Natasha said, "I felt sad, angry, and defeated. But I also felt free. I got excited because I realized that now there were other paths to parenthood that I could pursue."

Not everyone feels that excitement, though. And not everyone will want to pursue a different path to parenthood; some will prefer to be childfree. But please be careful not to cling to treatment in order to avoid facing the disappointment you will inevitably feel—the loss of your reproductive dreams. Only by facing your loss, as Paul did, will you gain a sense of closure.

Yet your work is not done. You need to honor your decision to stop. It is an emotional and complicated process to come to terms with not having a biological child. Even at this crossroads in your reproductive story, you may still have choices to face: depending on your medical situation, you may be considering donor technology or surrogacy, or feel ready to move onto adoption, or decide to remain childfree.

Coming to a mutual decision, finding something that works for both of you, and reaching the same conclusion at the same time can prove to be hard work. In the next chapter, we will explore the issues you may face as you proceed individually and as a couple to rewrite your reproductive stories.

Eleven

A New Ending, a New Beginning:
Rewriting Your Reproductive Story

You've been poked, prodded, medicated, discussed. You've fought, cried, struggled, grieved, and made sacrifices. Your self-esteem has been pummeled, your sense of yourself has been muddled, and your marriage has been stretched to the limit. Finally you've said, "Enough!" If only it stopped there. No sooner do you declare that you're done trying to have a biological child than another question forms itself: *What do we do now?*

At this pivotal point in your reproductive story, you and your partner are faced with more life-altering choices. You may decide to pursue parenthood through donor technology, surrogacy, or adoption, or you may choose to remain childfree. With any of these choices, you still must grieve what you have lost to clear the way for your new experience—with or without children. With each, you must rethink your reproductive story, decide what are the most important elements in it for you and your partner, and then rewrite your story to incorporate these changes.

Your story will not be the same as you originally anticipated—

that has become painfully clear—and no matter what path you choose, it will have its joys and challenges. But whether you become a parent or not, your reproductive story continues to unfold.

How do you figure out what's right for you? What if one day you are sure you want to adopt, yet the next day you think it would be better to be childfree? Or you find an egg donor, but your partner doesn't like your choice? What if you get scared and change your mind midstream? In this chapter, we discuss how the ending you are facing means new beginnings, what options are available to you, and how you can decide what will work best for you and your partner.

As sad as it is that a chapter of your reproductive story is ending, remember that you are at the threshold of a new beginning, and this new chapter of pursuing parenthood or not holds untold possibilities.

What Do We Do Next?

Couples vary in how they approach decisions of what to do next. Some begin to consider other options even as they try one final procedure for a biological child. They need to have their plan B in motion before they can bring themselves to stop treatment. This eases their anxiety about losing more time as they actively prepare for whatever comes next. When couples overlap these pages of their story, it may also soften the pain of giving up their dreams of having a biological child.

Ella and her husband Brett began researching adoption even as they tried one last IVF cycle. "I don't want to waste another minute," said Ella. "I will feel awful when the IVF doesn't work, especially if we are not prepared to move on. We've been at this too long. I'm tired of being sad. We need to be parents."

But not every couple has the next step in mind, and it does not always have to be decided immediately. It's okay to catch your breath and reflect on the trials you have been through. Often, couples need time to research—and soul search—what is right for them before they make their next move. "Of course, I've thought about IVF," Cliff said. "But before I can look into it, we need to finish this last IUI. And if it doesn't work, we're going to need some down time. We can't take on anything more right now."

It's important to realize that ending infertility treatment aimed at producing your own biological child is yet another loss. Sometimes, if you jump too quickly to the next treadmill, whatever that may be, you may bypass the need to respect and grieve how *this* chapter of your reproductive story ends. Yes, this can be painful and sad, but you need to reflect and accept this loss in order to move forward. Some couples, who have been grieving all along, may be ready to explore their options right away. But if you are burnt out from treatment, it may not be the best time to decide what to do. Talk to each other to discover whether you need to take a break before you decide what's next, or whether you feel ready to proceed.

To Parent or Not to Parent

To be a parent or not, that is the question you are facing now. And it is a complicated one, even though you've been pursuing that goal for so long. At this crossroads in your reproductive story, the answer isn't always clear.

As we discussed in chapter 10, knowing what is vital to your reproductive story and, of course, knowing your medical options will help you sift through the options of post-infertility treatment. Donor technology, surrogacy, and adoption can provide wonderful opportunities to infertile couples who long to become parents. This major change in your reproductive story, like all the others, must be grieved, but if parenthood is what you seek, the rewards can be boundless. It is all part of the process of rewriting your story, and the more prepared and aware you can be of all of your different feelings, the more fulfilling your alternate road to parenthood will be.

Here we raise some issues regarding each of these options, so you can consider and discuss them ahead of time. None of these concerns is insurmountable, but we want to emphasize how important it is to understand the options and talk things out at every stage of the process.

Donor Technology

If you want to experience pregnancy and birth, even if the child is not genetically connected to both of you, you may consider trying an IVF cycle with donor eggs, donor sperm, or donated embryos.

As much as donor technology may fulfill your reproductive dreams, the fact remains that the baby will have a biological connection to one parent, but not to the other. (Unless you are using donor embryos, in which case neither of you will have a genetic connection with the child.) The baby will not be biologically both of yours. This is a very real loss and every person who uses a donor must come to terms with it.

Some people worry they will not feel as attached to the baby if it's not "theirs," while others worry that the biological parent will somehow feel more authority or "ownership" over the baby. Of course, these ideas are feelings, not facts. But it is essential that you acknowledge and discuss these worries up front, in order to clarify how you both feel.

When choosing a donor, consider the pros and cons of using a known or anonymous donor. When a sister, brother, or other relative offers to be a donor, this is a complex gift. On the one hand, you'll have a genetic connection to the baby, as well as full access to family and medical history. On the other hand, both you and the donor have reproductive stories—and those can conflict. Will long-hidden sibling rivalries resurface when you don't expect it? Will your sibling or relative be comfortable being the aunt or uncle to your baby, not its parent? How might the rest of your family react?

Using an anonymous donor raises different questions. How do you choose one? Do you base your decision on how the donor looks? On their educational background or academic test scores? On their ethnic background or health history? The information that you receive from the donor or agency may be limited. If possible, obtain an in-depth psychological evaluation of your potential donor. Don't be afraid to ask questions about difficult-to-discuss matters of physical and mental health history either, including drug use or mental or emotional disorders.

Surrogacy

If carrying a child is not a possibility but passing on your genes or your partner's genes is vital to you, then using a surrogate may be a solution. In "gestational" surrogacy, an infertile couple contracts with a woman who carries embryos created by the infertile couple's egg and sperm (or in some cases donor egg and sperm). So-called "traditional" surrogacy also exists—that's when the surrogate is artificially inseminated with the father's sperm or donor sperm. As with egg donation, the surrogate can either be someone the couple knows or not, eliciting concerns similar to those we described above.

What kind of relationship do you have with a surrogate? How involved in her life do you get, during the pregnancy and afterward? To what degree can you dictate her lifestyle choices during gestation—for example, what she eats or whether she exercises? How will *she* feel about giving birth to a child and then giving it up? Again, the answers to these complicated questions vary from case to case, and situation to situation, but these questions need to be considered.

Both the surrogate's and the intended parents' expectations about the nature of their relationship, during the pregnancy and afterward, need careful attention. "At one point during the pregnancy, Josie, our surrogate, seemed upset," said Olivia. Olivia wasn't sure what was going on; she and her husband had tried to respect Josie's privacy and not intrude. "At first we worried that she was becoming too attached to the baby. Then we realized that what she needed was to feel closer to us, which was great because it was hard not to call her every day! Once we focused more attention on her, instead of just the baby, she felt better, and so did we."

Adoption

If what is most important to your reproductive story is becoming parents and a family, adoption might be the right choice.

Adoption has been a wonderful path to parenthood for many years—there is a baby at the end of the road. Even so, there are many decisions to be made about which type of adoption to pursue, and the process itself involves logistical hurdles, emotional pitfalls, and sometimes some risk.

There are many questions to consider. Which adoption path do you want to pursue? Do you want to adopt domestically? Privately or through an agency? Are you willing to adopt an older child, a child of a different ethnicity, or a child whose birth mother smokes or uses drugs or alcohol? Do you want an open or closed adoption? Most domestic adoptions today are open, meaning that adopted children know who their biological parents are, but how open a situation are you comfortable with? How much contact do you want to have with the birth parents after the baby is yours? And then there is the question that every adoptive parent worries about: will the birth parents change their minds?

More questions arise. Do you want to adopt internationally? Which country? How long are you willing to wait? How much travel are you willing to undertake? What health issues are you most concerned about? International adoption can involve lots of paperwork plus waits before you are matched with a child.

How do you even begin to decide all these things? One of the biggest obstacles for many couples is that once again they feel hopeless, with the control in someone else's hands. Information helps—but the direct, personal kind is the most important. We have found that people have an easier time considering and coming to terms with the idea of adoption when they know more people who have done it, or when adoptions have occurred in their own families. Talking to other parents who have obtained or

added to their families through adoption gives you firsthand information. Just as important, you'll see how families with adopted
children can work, thus quelling anxieties you may feel. Bonnie
found it relatively easy to contemplate adoption when she and Ser-
gio were faced with infertility treatment that was not working, because one of her older brothers had adopted two children.

What's most important to remember, even if there can be hassles with adoption, is that you *will* get to be a parent. Carol and
Bryan adopted a baby after two years of treatment. "We thought
long and hard about it all," Carol said, "and then one day it hit
me—I won't have to go through all this anxiety and medical stuff
anymore. I thought, so what if I'm not good at getting pregnant,
somebody else can do that for me. Someone else can do the work
of pregnancy and I'll do the work of parenting. And now that we
have our son, it's a job I love."

Choosing to be Childfree

Some couples realize that if they can't have a biological child, they
would rather not have a child at all. "We've been emotionally
whipped by infertility," Audrey said. "The thought of trying to
have a child another way is too overwhelming. We're done. We've
decided to remain a family of two."

After so much time trying to have a baby, the decision to remain childfree is by no means an easy one. But it's an important
choice to consider. Deciding not to have children can open up
new doors, as you pursue other dreams and interests: maybe to
travel, volunteer, or change careers.

This is of course a complicated decision, and most couples who
decide to remain childfree have moments of pain and doubt. Just

because you have decided on a childfree life doesn't mean you don't think about the "what ifs" from time to time. Even when you make a thoroughly considered decision to not have children and you mourn this loss, certain events in life may reawaken a sense of longing or regret. This is to be expected. Remember, too, that grieving is a twofold process: you must cope with the loss at the same time as you rebuild a life for yourself without the person or dream that you've lost.

How Do We Know What's Right for Us?

Sometimes it helps to imagine what your life will be like in five or ten years from now—with or without children. Will you have regrets? Will you berate yourself for making the wrong choice?

Eilene, thirty-nine years old and single, wanted to be a parent even though she wasn't currently in a significant relationship, so she decided to use donor sperm for her IUIs. "I never thought I'd be a single parent, but I know I want to be a mother, and I can't wait for 'Mr. Right' anymore."

It was helpful for Eilene to project into the future. "I could be fifty and have a ten-year-old, or I could be alone and miss out on it all." For her, imagining life without the experience of motherhood felt too empty, so in spite of the difficulties of being a single parent, she opted to move forward with a sperm donor.

Mike and Nadine had been through four IVFs and numerous IUIs over the past four years. When their doctor suggested they might need to turn to donor eggs or surrogacy, the couple took some time to think. Both imagined their own futures and found satisfaction in their careers: Nadine, 40, was a middle-school teacher, Mike, 45, a computer programmer who also coached ten-

nis at Nadine's school. "We realized that life is pretty good 'as is,'"
Nadine said. "We've got a great relationship, and are always on the
go. Our lives would radically change if we had a baby. It's not that
I don't think about it at times—I'd be lying if I said I never get
wistful. But we're both very involved with kids; I'm with them
every day. And even though it's not the same as having your own,
it does have its advantages." Nadine laughed as she added, "For instance—they go home at the end of the day! And with some of
these middle schoolers, that's a really good thing." Taking stock of
their relationship and their life together, they decided to "count
their blessings," as they put it, and be childfree.

Just as you researched your treatment options, it is important to
investigate your options at this stage as well. Many organizations
and clinics offer workshops on adoption, donor technology, surrogacy, and living childfree. Talk with others who have gone through
the process to help answer your questions. Many physicians and
clinics also offer consultations and/or seminars to review what
might be best for you, with regard to donor technology or surrogacy. The Internet is another resource.

After you evaluate your choices, you may still feel ambivalent.
It's normal to settle on one possibility and then find that your feelings change overnight.

Other People's Two Cents

Do keep in mind that everyone and their uncle will opine about
what you should do next. Once again well-intentioned suggestions
can be infuriating and intrusive. The classic line is: "Just adopt,
then you'll get pregnant" but the truth is that most couples who do
adopt don't get pregnant, right away or ever.

If you choose a less traditional way to build a family, or decide not to have children, you may encounter raised eyebrows and unsolicited advice. When Marlene approached her sister-in-law Risa for support as she considered egg donation, she was hurt by Risa's response. "I can't imagine using an egg donor," said Risa, who has three biological children. "It would be strange to have a baby that wasn't mine."

Similarly, Alyssa's friends were horrified that she wanted to remain childfree. "Everyone had an opinion about what we should do next," Alyssa said. "But when I mentioned that we were content the way we are—that we had made peace with ourselves about going through life without a child—some of my friends became indignant. One implied that we were being selfish if we didn't adopt."

If people offend you with their opinions, you can reply: "Thanks for your input, but this is what's right for us." Or if someone asks if you have kids when you've decided to be childfree, you can simply answer, "No," or if you want to go into more detail you can say, "We would have liked to, but it didn't work out."

The problem is you may not yet know what's right for you. All this pressure comes at a time when you have already been through the emotional mill. And the choices and decisions you need to make at this point are some of the most challenging—and the most personal.

What if Your Rewrites Have Different Plots?

What happens if you and your partner don't agree on how to proceed? After struggling with infertility for so long, couples often have different ideas about when to stop and what to do next. Your individual reproductive stories may veer in different directions at this pivotal time.

Patricia wanted to use an egg donor, since for her, the experience of pregnancy and birth was paramount. "Even if I'm not biologically related, I know the baby would feel like mine if I carried it for nine months. That's more important to me than DNA. I want to know what it's like to nurture a life inside me."

But her husband, Rob, felt uncomfortable. "The best situation would be if the baby was biologically related to both of us," he said. "But if it can't be both, I feel it should be neither. I'm worried about what might happen down the line, if she feels that the baby is more mine than hers because of a biological connection. I know that's how I'd feel if the situation was reversed."

What do you do if you find yourself at an impasse with your partner? After all you've been through, tensions can flare again when it feels as though your partner is blocking you from your dreams. If you think of your partner as a gate-keeper, then resentment is sure to factor into how you feel. What you don't want is for one person to give in to the other's wishes, only to harbor anger and bitterness in years to come. And you don't want to be stuck in a control struggle over what to do.

Now, more than ever, you need to be open and honest about your reproductive story and how you see your rewrite. And you need to listen and consider your partner's story as well. Weigh the plusses and minuses of each side and let your partner know what is important to you and why. If you understand the meaning of these reproductive decisions from each other's perspective, you can have greater empathy for each other.

If there is a conflict, it can help to remember what you do agree on—that is, that you both want to have a family—and work backward from there. Both Patricia and Rob knew they wanted a child; their impasse was over how to get there. When Rob described to Patricia how he would feel if the situation was reversed—if he wasn't biologically connected to the child—Patricia understood his fears. And she explained to Rob that she would love their baby, no matter its origins, and she reassured him they were equal partners no matter what.

After discussing each other's points of view, Patricia and Rob both softened. They agreed that he would research egg donors and she would research adoption; they would both learn more about their options and then use that knowledge to balance their emotional concerns.

These are by no means easy discussions or easy compromises. If you find yourself stuck and getting nowhere—for example, you want to pursue parenthood and your partner does not—consider finding a therapist who can help mediate disputes. Remember, you've been emotionally worn down by infertility, but you do have choices. Your partner isn't your prisoner. Recognizing your choices and deciding what to do next can be challenging, but it isn't impossible.

Sadly, some couples break up when their reproductive stories don't mesh. This sometimes occurs in younger couples who haven't been together as long. In relationships whose primary goal is starting a family, a partner who has the main infertility problem may be left behind. But more often, we see couples who struggle with how damaged they feel and with the rage that accompanies repeated loss but has nowhere to go. In such cases, self-blame and wounds to each partner's narcissism are replaced by convictions that the *other* partner is really the bad one. Making that assumption, an individual may feel that the bad feelings can be escaped by escaping the relationship.

But one of the tragedies of infertility is that most of the pain is internal, and not caused by the other person, and can only be prevented, coped with, or healed by the means we have tried to describe in this book.

Rebuilding Your Sexual Relationship

After all the tension between the two of you brought on by infertility, you may even find renewed romance when you set about rewriting your story. Following years of treatment and timed, task-oriented sex, it can be a relief to enjoy each other again. It may take time to rekindle your relationship; intimacy may remind you of all your failed attempts. Your weakened sense of both your physical and emotional self may interfere with your relationship, sexually or otherwise. But just as you have the opportunity to rethink your own identity, you and your partner can reevaluate this next phase of your life together.

The reestablishment of sexual intimacy is important even after childbirth without infertility, and is all the more crucial after infertility. It may take time, but we advise couples to commit to reconnecting in this way. Pleasure and intimacy of this kind can go a long way toward healing the wounds you have both experienced over the long and arduous course of infertility treatment.

Your Ongoing Story

No matter what choice you make after you stop infertility treatment, your reproductive story continues to unfold. Your first

choice, having your own biological offspring, is not possible, and
the alternatives made possible by modern medicine may or may
not be right for you.

Knowing what is the next best step for you and your partner
takes time. Without meaning to sound like a broken record, our
message to you is that there are no right or wrong choices at this
juncture in your reproductive story. The beauty of the reproductive story is that it can be written and rewritten as you go through
your life. Your infertility trauma will never be completely erased—
it will always be a part of you—but it will be only a part, a single
chapter, in the story of your life.

Twelve

Parenting After Infertility:
Singing Your Lullabies at Last

I have never felt more exhausted in my life. We waited years for a baby—and when Molly arrived we were more than thrilled! She's a joy and a delight and I am so happy—I know she's a wonderful child, smart and into everything—but she's also a handful. I'm so stressed about being a good mother that I can't completely let go and enjoy her. I worry that we are spoiling her, and then again, I worry that we are not doing enough for her. Plus Jeff and I disagree about parenting issues and we've been arguing. She is a strong-willed little girl and has a temper—how can we deal with her temper when we can't cope with our own? After struggling with infertility, it feels unfair to be struggling again now that we finally have a child.

—Louise, adoptive mother after four years of infertility

Infertility is a long, arduous road, with countless moments of hope and disappointment. For many couples, the struggle finally pays off . . . you have a baby! Whether it's through successful medical treatment, egg or sperm donation, surrogacy, or adoption, a child has finally entered your life.

Your journey to parenthood has been fraught with loss, pain, anxiety, stress, and enormous expense. You and your partner have been through the gauntlet together, cried, fought, hated each other, loved each other, and drawn closer than ever before. Throughout your ordeal, your reproductive story has been thrown off-track, twisted and turned, and has been written and rewritten. Finally after all the turmoil, you can sing the lullabies you have dreamed of for so long.

As Nathan, a new adoptive father of Benjamin, following six years of infertility, says: "Even when I am exhausted, or Ben won't stop screaming, or I'm changing a dirty diaper, I can't believe how lucky I feel. I never imagined I could love someone this much. It makes it all worthwhile."

Having a baby in your arms soothes many of infertility's wounds. But becoming a parent after infertility can also bring unexpected emotions. Feeling depressed, anxious, or exhausted after a baby arrives is quite normal—for every new parent. But when these feelings occur after the long haul of infertility, couples may become alarmed by them. We have often heard people fret: "How could I possibly feel bad about being a parent after I've struggled so hard to get here?"

While having a baby profoundly affects your future, it does not erase your past. Having been through so much, it can be confusing to feel both ecstatic as well as depressed. In this chapter we discuss:

- the many complex emotions of a pregnancy post-infertility
- the complications that infertile couples often face because of high-risk pregnancies, prematurity, or multiple births
- how the reality of having a child often differs from the fantasized baby

- how to deal with your negative feelings: just because you fought long and hard to have a child doesn't mean you are protected from difficult postpartum reactions
- the reparative effects of finally having a child to nurture and love

Pregnancy After Infertility

Celia, who just turned forty, is pregnant after her fourth IVF. "It took five very long years, but we finally did it! When the pregnancy test came back positive, I burst into tears. I was thrilled, but at the same time panicked. I worry every day that something bad is going to happen," she said.

Many couples who have gone through infertility echo Celia's fears. After so much going wrong, it's hard to believe things could possibly go right. Some couples feel cautiously optimistic; others are on edge throughout the pregnancy, wondering "when the other shoe might drop." Waiting for pending test results may be high-stress times. "We were relieved when we heard the heartbeat," Celia continued. "But then my infertility doctor said I should see my regular ob/gyn. He said everything looked great and I didn't need him anymore. That was a shock. 'You mean, I'm normal?' I asked. I couldn't believe it."

Not only was the pregnancy "normal" but her feelings were as well. It's hard to trust your body after it hasn't worked the way you expected it to. Celia needed frequent reassurance from her doctors. "When I saw my daughter on the ultrasound, it started to become real to me. And when the amnio results came back indicating all was well, I started to relax," she said.

Women who have not experienced infertility describe the attachment they feel toward their baby in utero. But women who have struggled with infertility often remain emotionally removed. Staying detached is a way to protect yourself from yet another loss. Toby, who miscarried at fourteen weeks, was pregnant again two years later. "Even after I passed into my third trimester," she said, "I didn't believe it was real. About two weeks before my son was born, the doctor measured me and said, 'We're there.' What an emotional moment that was. Only then did I begin to believe this was really going to happen."

The Additional Challenge of a High-Risk Pregnancy

Many infertile couples face complicated, high-risk pregnancies and premature births, especially if they are carrying twins or more. These events can represent still more blows to your self-esteem. You may feel you are to blame if something goes wrong, just as you felt during infertility. Further, the demands of caring for multiple or premature babies can be very different from the scenario that you have dreamed of for so long, leaving you feeling once again that your reproductive story is off course.

If you end up giving birth early, for whatever reason, you may feel tense and guilty. Women often wonder what they could have done to prevent a premature delivery, as if this were in their control. These feelings can arise for anyone who has had a preemie, but may be especially difficult for someone who has struggled with infertility. After so much time spent trying to take charge of the infertility, you are in yet another situation where you feel responsible for things going wrong. Once again, though, this is a *feeling;* even though it is your body, the reality is that labor pains and birth are not in your control.

Cynthia, pregnant after trying for four years, was put on bed rest in her sixth month. She delivered her daughter eight weeks early. "I was so thankful and delighted to have my daughter, especially after all the trials we went through to get her. Then, when she was in the hospital's preemie unit, we were beside ourselves, hoping she would be all right. But even though she came so early, she pulled through."

Cynthia, delighted that her daughter was thriving and catching up developmentally, still remained upset about the pregnancy, as if somehow she didn't do it right. She was surprised by her feelings that the pregnancy ended too soon. "I feel as if I somehow missed out—or like I didn't quite finish what I was supposed to," she said. "I have some brand-new maternity clothes that I didn't get to wear. It feels strange to be down because of this, but it was so hard to get pregnant in the first place and now I feel like I didn't do the pregnancy right either."

The feeling of "not getting it right"—having difficulty with the pregnancy—was yet another blow to Cynthia's self-esteem. In her case, she knew that the chances of her getting pregnant again and having another child were slim. She felt that the pregnancy she did have would be her only chance. It took some time to sort through her feelings and realize that having her pregnancy end early was another way her reproductive story had been altered. Once she was able to realize that this too was a loss, she could focus on what she does "do right," like caring for her infant in her new role as a mom.

If you experience a high-risk pregnancy, chances are you will be in a coping mode, as you were going through infertility treatment, until you and your baby are out of the woods. You may think that the celebrations will begin as soon as everything resolves medically.

But keep in mind that often people only experience their shock or grief after the crisis has passed.

The Reality of a Baby Versus the Fantasy of One

When a baby enters your life, however it arrives, a new and different struggle begins. The reality of parenthood sets in, complete with two A.M. feedings, crying, burping, spit-up, and dirty diapers. All new parents are overwhelmed by how difficult, unpredictable, and exhausting caring for an infant can be.

You may relish the physical work of caring for an infant, and feel grateful to finally be handling parenthood's hassles. Yet it's not always easy. Having longed for a baby for so long, and fantasized about how wonderful it would be, you may not be prepared for some of the challenges, and may find it hard to accept the negative feelings that sometimes accompany them.

Ellen, who had several miscarriages and a failed IVF before deciding to use donor eggs, was delighted when she found out that three eggs implanted. "I remember thinking, 'Triplets, what fun!' But now I don't know which end is up," she said. "As soon as I get one settled, another one starts crying. I know I should be thankful; how can I complain after all we've been through? But this is really hard. I feel as if I've gone from one battlefield to another with no rest in between."

As we've noted above, every new parent struggles with discomfort and self-doubt in the transition to parenthood. And every new parent must incorporate their fantasized expectations of parenthood with reality. But since you have fought so hard for this baby and gone through so much, you may be even less prepared for the range of emotions you're confronting. Having focused for so long on becoming parents, your expectations are especially high, not only of your baby, but of yourself. Not only do you expect to have an absolutely wonderful baby, you also feel pressure to be a perfect parent. This can be an enormous burden and interfere with your ability to enjoy your baby.

So what can you do? Remember that when you become a parent after infertility, you are working to heal your emotional wounds at the same time you have a new job as a parent. As we explained in chapter 5, it's normal for parents to view their children as narcissistic extensions of themselves; we all want to see our babies—and ourselves—as wonderful. But infertility trauma batters your self-esteem and inflicts narcissistic injury. If you are trying to be a perfect parent, you may be compensating for the damage to your self-esteem that infertility can inflict. As always, it is crucial to separate infertility from who you are as a parent. Just as it is unfair to expect your baby to be perfect, it is unfair to expect yourself to be perfect either.

Postpartum Reactions after Infertility

After traveling on the infertility roller coaster for seven years, Cathy is confounded by her mixed feelings. "I don't understand what is happening to me," she said. "I am upset all the time. I love my baby and I want to be a good mother, but I feel more depressed now than ever. How can I be depressed when having a baby is all I've wanted for the longest time? How can I be a good mother when I feel this bad?"

Cathy believes she is not entitled to feel full of doubt or overwhelmed. But in fact, these are normal, expected reactions for new parents. And going through infertility doesn't mean that you are automatically protected from having the postpartum blues, depression, or other reactions. Even couples who adopt may have complicated postpartum reactions. It's not just hormonal shifts that cause postpartum disorders.

"I got so upset with myself the other day," said Lacey, a new mother after six years of infertility. "I was trying to get some housework done—the laundry was stacked up a mile high—and Noah wouldn't go down for a nap. He cried and cried. I didn't know what was wrong and I didn't know what to do. I couldn't comfort him or get him settled down. What upset me was how angry it made me. Me! Of all people to get angry with my baby! After I waited six years for him!"

If you find yourself suddenly feeling upset with your baby—over anything from having to change yet another diaper to having difficulty getting the baby to sleep—your anxiety and guilt over getting annoyed may make you feel inadequate. Please be reassured that every new parent needs to adjust to the demands of a new baby, and that a range of negative feelings is a natural part of this process.

Postpartum depression, anxiety, and other conditions can happen and need to be taken seriously. They can come as a shock and another blow to your self-esteem. You might want to find a postpartum support group where you can talk about your feelings and compare notes with other new moms. It's comforting to know that other women, whether they have had infertility or not, worry that they are not doing motherhood "perfectly" and may be overwhelmed by the demands of new parenthood.

Many women resist getting the help they need, especially after infertility. After so much time spent feeling vulnerable and out of control, it can feel like a cruel joke to continue feeling the same way. You may feel ashamed that you can't do this as you expected you would—after all, you went to great lengths to have this baby. Remember, however, that this is an adjustment period. It's normal that lots of feelings will emerge now that your baby is finally here.

On the other hand, if you are completely overwhelmed with emotion after your baby arrives, find yourself crying all the time, can't get out of bed, or feel that you can't care for your baby, you must seek professional help. A period of mild blue moods is relatively common in the first two weeks or so after your child has arrived, but these kinds of more pronounced and persistent signs require serious attention. Your baby's pediatrician or your ob/gyn should be able to refer you to a therapist who can help you better understand what you are experiencing and take appropriate measures to treat it.

Signs for Postpartum Depression
Seeking professional help is necessary:

- if you find yourself in tears most days or can't get out of bed or feel hopeless and helpless
- if you are so anxious that you can't leave your baby for a moment (even though you know she/he is safe)
- if you have other worries which affect your sleep or cause you to obsess
- if you feel as though you might hurt your baby, or can't take care of him/her
- if you feel as though you might hurt yourself
- if any of these symptoms last for more than a couple of weeks.

Stored-up Grief

For infertile couples, the arrival of a baby, through birth or adoption, may be the first time in the grueling infertility process that you let down your guard. Only after you have a child can you comprehend and grieve the ordeal you have been through. It is not that you are unhappy about being a parent or feel dissatisfied with your child—far from it. It's that now, after the nightmare has finally ended, the grief can—and does—come pouring out. So along with the challenges of new parenthood, you may begin to release all the tension and grief that has been pent-up for years. Couples are often taken by surprise by these feelings that arise well after the difficult experience they've been through. But delayed grief is to be expected. It can be helpful to refer to chapter 8 to understand and deal with such emotions.

The Twosome Becomes a Threesome

You may have imagined that, as your twosome becomes a threesome, everything now would finally be just right. But couples sometimes struggle more with their transition into actual parenthood than they had anticipated. Roles change dramatically when a child enters your life. One of you may have stopped working, while the other is working more. You may have moved into a new neighborhood, and you may be exhausted by constant caretaking demands. Although marital stress is normal and to be expected during such a significant life change, couples who have been through infertility may once again feel that there's something wrong when they experience it.

New fathers may feel a special conflict when they finally become parents after infertility. If they have coped with the trauma by becoming the support person for their wives, they may have hoped that they will "get her back" when the infertility is finally behind them. Instead, the focus has shifted from him taking care of her to both of them taking care of the baby. A new dad may continue to feel quite alone—or even more alone—with a sense that his feelings *still* don't matter after a baby is born. While every new father must deal with the recognition that his wife is now someone's mother, this shift may be especially painful for men who have gone through the trauma of infertility and who have felt inadequate or emotionally isolated from their wives for long periods of time.

Similarly, a new mother may struggle with the double burdens of taking care of her baby and trying to regain her equilibrium following infertility. She may continue to feel a high need for support from her husband, at the same time that she wants to feel healthy and independent once again. Couples need to stay attuned to these issues and find a balance between taking care of their own needs, paying attention to each other, and nurturing their baby.

Members of the "Club" at Last

Although becoming a parent will not erase the trauma you've experienced, it does help you to begin healing some of the wounds caused by your infertility experience. So long excluded from the "club," you can now breathe a sigh of relief; you finally have joined the ranks of your contemporaries, your elders, and what has sometimes seemed like the rest of the world, as parents.

"After being an infertility patient for seven years, I was beginning to think that there was no other way to be," said Wendy. "Now my only visits to doctors' offices are for well-baby checkups. It feels so good to be 'normal' again."

When you are finally a parent after infertility, the blows to your self-esteem inflicted by the trauma can be replaced by a sense of self-worth in your new role as mother or father. "I feel like people are treating me differently," said Toni, who adopted a baby girl domestically after five years of infertility. "It's almost as if I got a promotion at work with a new title to go with my new responsibilities. I am now a 'mom.'" Toni's feeling that she has been "promoted" partly reflects how diminished and awful she felt about herself before, rather than changes in how her colleagues react to her. What matters most is that she has regained a healing sense of pride and now feels better about herself.

Many new parents relish their newfound sense of belonging. No longer do they feel awkward when gathering with friends or family, or when meeting new people. No longer do they have to field questions about having kids. Closed doors are now reopening. "I remember taking Zack to the park for the first time," said Jocelyn, 38, who had become pregnant by IVF after four years of infertility. "He was tucked into his Snugli as we walked around the playground. I felt so proud. I met another woman there who had a four-month-old. Although she looked younger than me, and I had been through so much, somehow, at that moment, it didn't matter. As we talked shop, we were both just moms, and it felt good to be accepted as one."

Nathan, Benjamin's adoptive father, used to dread going to his folks' for the holidays. "It was hard to enjoy it—so much of the focus was on my nieces and nephews, as it should be—but we felt like the 'odd couple.' This year everything feels different. Having Ben has completely changed our perspective. It is good to feel a part of it all again."

Back on Track in Life

The healing that comes with becoming a parent is not just about feeling proud of your accomplishment or regaining a sense of belonging. When you have a baby, you may feel relief at being back on your developmental track, after being thrown off course by infertility. Now your reproductive story and your sense of your adult self may once again unfold in the way that you had hoped. As a parent, you shift from the role of child to that of parent, and can forge a new bond with your parents as peers. You may gain a greater understanding of them as people, as well as of your own childhood. As Annie, who conceived on her third IUI, said, "After Lily was born, my mother and I became much closer than before. It's like we had more in common now. We could compare notes as two mothers and feel a kinship."

Just as things feel different between you and your parents once you have a child, your relationship with your siblings may also shift, especially if they had children before you. Kay, who had a baby by egg donation, reflected on this. "My younger sister had two children while I was going through infertility treatment. Although she was very supportive, it was still very tense. It was like she had become the 'big sister,'" she said. "Since I've had Natalie, we talk to each other nearly every day and it feels like we are sisters again."

Your relationship with your partner also has a much-needed chance to heal. You can regain a sense of progress and being back on track as a couple, just as you do as individuals. You will get to know each other in new ways, as parents, when your shared dream has been achieved. While it can be challenging, it is also exciting and refreshing to a relationship that has been through the mill.

What if You Want Another Baby?

People whose reproductive stories have unfolded smoothly may have a distinct feeling of completeness when they have had the children they wanted, whether it was one, two, or five. But not everyone feels this way, even if they have not gone through infertility. Very often, people grieve when they realize that there are not going to be any more babies—it can be bittersweet to close the chapter on that part of life. Rose, a woman in her late sixties who has three grown daughters, said, "Two of my girls are pregnant right now, and it's the craziest thing—last night I had a dream that I wanted another baby too! I was angry with my husband when I woke up because he had wanted to stop at three kids—even though that had been my choice also. I guess you never feel really 'done.'"

If you have gone through infertility and have finally been able to become a parent even to one child, you—and others—may presume that it means everything is now as it should be, that your reproductive story is now set right. But what if you had hoped to have several children? What if you have a son and want a daughter too? Becoming a parent following infertility does not necessarily mean that your reproductive story is over. If you have secondary infertility, you continue to deal with painful situations.

"Wow, you guys are such great parents—why won't you have more kids?" someone at work might exclaim, as if this were purely a matter of choice. If you had hoped to have more than one child but can't, you must once again grieve the lost parts of your story. Remember that this may always be a sensitive spot for you. Again it helps to keep some responses in your back pocket, so you are prepared if someone says something thoughtless. Humor, with a little sarcasm, can help: you might retort, "Well, you're a great wife to your husband, why don't you get a second one?" Or you might reply, "Thank you for your kind thoughts. We really do love our son. But sometimes having more just isn't meant to be." Or, "You never know what a person's story is, do you?"

Unused Embryos

What to do with unused embryos is a question that many couples grapple with. You may not know what to do with them if your family is complete, or you are not in a position medically or financially to use them. While some couples feel no conflict about disposing of embryos, others have a harder time. Some couples feel an enormous attachment to unused embryos: "They're my babies."

Some people resolve this dilemma by donating their unused embryos. Isabel, after giving birth to twins, knew that she did not want any more children. She decided to give her embryos up for "adoption" and donated them. "It feels better to me," she said. "Like I can find some good in this whole nightmare by helping someone else have a family."

Whatever you choose to do as a couple, you must both feel comfortable about your decision. What is right for some may not be right for others; the guidelines to these decisions come from how you feel.

What Do You Tell Your Child?

When you become a parent after infertility, you must decide what, when, and how to tell your child about his or her origins. How you choose to handle this will depend largely on your perception of your child's ability to understand what you tell him/her, and at what age.

If a child is the result of donor technology or adoption, most parents feel that he or she has a right to know his/her medical and family history, but they wonder when they should share this information. "I want to tell my son about his roots," said Angela, "but I don't think he is old enough to understand. But if I don't tell him soon, I'm afraid he will be upset with me for withholding the truth. I worry that he'll think I have lied about other things too and not trust me anymore."

Although Angela is trying to be sensitive to her son's feelings, it is important to remember that parents withhold all sorts of information from their children until they feel the child is old enough to handle it. Parents make these decisions throughout a child's growing up, whether it is explaining the facts of life to a little one, or revealing whether or not you ever tried drugs to a teenager. There is an appropriate time and context in which to talk to kids about all sorts of topics, and information about their conception is no exception.

Several points are significant here: first is that you and your partner come to an agreement on how and when to talk to your child about his or her history. It's not urgent when they are infants, so you can take some time to think it over, or even discuss it with other parents you meet who are in similar situations.

Second, it's important that your child learn of his or her birth circumstances from *you* rather than from someone else. This is a reason not to postpone the decision about what and when to tell for too long, because you can't predict or control what friends and relatives will say to your child.

Third, try to make sure the substance and timing of any explanations you offer your child fit their own concerns and developmental level, rather than reflect your own anxieties. We recommend that parents who are preparing to talk to their kids pause and examine not only what they are going to say, but also how they feel about saying it. Really strong feelings or overly elaborate explanations may mean you have residual feelings about the infertility experience, and those need to be separated from what your child really needs to hear.

When you talk to your child, be straightforward and matter of fact and tailor your explanation to match your child's age and level of understanding. During the conversation, watch for signals from your child about whether he or she wants and needs to know more details, or is satisfied with what you've said so far.

Kris, an infertile woman who became pregnant with donor sperm, told her son about this when he became interested in "where babies come from." She explained about the sperm and the egg and then added, "Sometimes, like with Dad, the sperm doesn't work very well. So to make you, we borrowed some." Lyle thought about this for a moment and then said, "Oh, but he's still my dad, right?" "Of course he is," said Kris, smiling inside and out.

The Never-ending Story

As with all aspects of your reproductive story, your experience of becoming a parent following infertility will be unique and highly personal. There will be times when the "lullabies" you sing feel fulfilling, and other times when you may feel frustrated that they are not being heard, either due to the clamoring of your baby or the emotional clamoring within your self. There will be joys and frustrations, successes and self-doubts. As always, be patient with yourselves as you traverse this new land called parenthood. Stay connected with yourself and with your partner, and continue to reflect and communicate.

Finally, as your child grows up, know that you will continue to work through your infertility trauma. You may not feel the trauma as intensely as you feel it today, but it will always be a part of you. Infertility is never something chosen, but it makes us take stock of our lives in profound and unexpected ways.

Epilogue

You have reached the end of this book, but your reproductive story is far from over. Having walked in your shoes, we, the authors, know that the experience of your infertility will be woven into the fabric of your life as your story unfolds, whether or not you have children.

We know, because although we all eventually became parents, we still relive the days, months, and years of our own infertility experiences. Sometimes the memories are vivid and painful, and we must rework them again whenever they come up. Janet remembers walking into her first support group meeting feeling like a loser, ashamed and demoralized. Martha and David still recall their shared struggles, the times they were able to help each other as well as the times when they couldn't, and just got by.

But as vivid as some memories remain for us, many others have faded. Like a collection of old photographs, they are at the bottom of the box, with new ones on top, the old images faded with time. When we revisit those memories, like looking at old pictures, we see how each of us, in different ways, has changed and grown from our experiences. Janet has become a person who now provides support to others, as she once received it. Dave and Martha stay attuned to each other's stories in ever deeper ways, while they help others discover their own inner narratives.

Most of all, we have learned an enormous amount about ourselves, and about the depth and complexity of human relationships. We have learned about the meaning of children to parents, parents to children, and the meaning of dreams, stories, and hopes to us all. Having known trauma and loss firsthand, we appreciate a little more both the joys and the tears we have felt raising our own children, and we have gained respect and admiration for others who are on these same journeys, with or without children.

You might not believe this now if you are in the middle of this tumultuous chapter of your story, but you will get through it. Right now your life, your plans, and your sense of self have been turned upside down. Your marriage has been under siege, and you have faced loss over and over. When we were in the midst of it all, we didn't believe we'd ever feel differently, but we do, and so will you.

Whether you are still involved in treatment, have become a parent through alternate means, or have decided to remain childfree, your infertility trauma will become but one strand in the fabric of your reproductive life. As you continue to live and rewrite your story in the times to come, we hope you will find peace.

Resources

American Infertility Association (AIA)
666 Fifth Ave. Ste. 278
New York, NY 10103
(888) 917-3777
e-mail: info@americaninfertility.org
Web site: www.americaninfertility.org

American Society for Reproductive Medicine (ASRM)
1209 Montgomery Highway
Birmingham, AL 35216-2809
(205) 978-5000
e-mail: asrm@asrm.org
Web site: www.asrm.org

Center for Loss in Multiple Birth, Inc. (CLIMB)
P.O. Box 91377
Anchorage, AK 99509
(907) 222-5321
e-mail: climb@pobox.alaska.net
Web site: www.climb-support.org

Center For Reproductive Psychology
11777 Bernardo Plaza Ct. Ste. 108
San Diego, CA 92128
(858) 576-3810
e-mail: support@reproductivepsych.org
Web site: www.ReproductivePsych.org

Empty Cradle
Web site: www.empty-cradle.com

The International Council on Infertility Information Dissemination
(INCIID)
P.O. Box 6838
Arlington, VA 22206
(703) 379-9178
Web site: www.inciid.org

National Hospice and Palliative Care Organization (NHPCO)
1700 Diagonal Rd. Ste. 625
Alexandria, VA 22314
(703) 837-1500
Web site: www.nhpco.org

Postpartum Support International (PSI)
927 N. Kellogg Ave.
Santa Barbara, CA 93111
(805) 967-7636
e-mail: PSIOffice@earthlink.net
Web site: www.postpartum.net

RESOLVE: The National Infertility Association
1310 Broadway
Somerville, MA 02144-1779
e-mail: info@resolve.org
Web site: www.resolve.org

SHARE Pregnancy and Infant Loss Support, Inc.
National Share Office
St. Joseph Health Center
300 First Capitol Dr.
St. Charles, MO 63301-2893
(800) 821-6819
e-mail: share@nationalshareoffice.com
Web site: www.nationalshareoffice.com

Index

About the Authors

Janet Jaffe, Ph.D., Martha Diamond, Ph.D., and David Diamond, Ph.D., are psychologists in private practice and are cofounders and codirectors of the Center for Reproductive Psychology in San Diego. They have presented nationally and internationally on the psychology of the reproductive process. A psychoanalyst, David is a faculty member of the California School of Professional Psychology (CSPP), at Alliant International University, where Martha and Janet also serve as instructors. David also leads the Reproductive Psychology Study Group at CSPP.

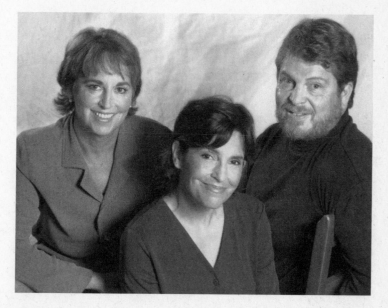

Martha Diamond, Janet Jaffe, and David Diamond. Photo by Rebecca Lawson